汉英对照

# 中医养生经典译丛

Chinese-English Translation of Traditional
Chinese Medicine Classics on Health Preservation

# 养性延命录

## Records on Health Preservation and Longevity

[南北朝] 陶弘景 撰

李成华 孔冉冉 孙慧明 主译

山东科学技术出版社

·济南·

**图书在版编目（CIP）数据**

养性延命录：汉英对照 /（南北朝）陶弘景撰；李成华，孔冉冉，孙慧明主译 . -- 济南：山东科学技术出版社，2023.3（2025.3 重印）

ISBN 978-7-5723-1498-8

Ⅰ . ①养…　Ⅱ . ①陶…　②李…　③孔…　④孙…　Ⅲ . ①养生（中医）- 中国 - 南朝时代 - 汉、英　Ⅳ . ① R212

中国国家版本馆 CIP 数据核字 (2023) 第 026610 号

# 养性延命录
YANGXING YANMING LU

责任编辑：马　祥　夏元枢
装帧设计：孙小杰

主管单位：山东出版传媒股份有限公司
出 版 者：山东科学技术出版社
　　　　　地址：济南市市中区舜耕路 517 号
　　　　　邮编：250003　电话：（0531）82098088
　　　　　网址：www.lkj.com.cn
　　　　　电子邮件：sdkj@sdcbcm.com
发 行 者：山东科学技术出版社
　　　　　地址：济南市市中区舜耕路 517 号
　　　　　邮编：250003　电话：（0531）82098067
印 刷 者：北京兰星球彩色印刷有限公司
　　　　　地址：北京市海淀区亮甲店 1 号
　　　　　邮编：100020　电话：（010）58411596

规格：16 开（170 mm×240 mm）
印张：6　字数：86 千
版次：2023 年 3 月第 1 版　印次：2025 年 3 月第 2 次印刷
定价：38.00 元

# 丛书序

中医学注重未病先防，倡导不治已病治未病，强调养生的重要性。自《黄帝内经》问世以来，华佗、张仲景、王冰、叶天士等历代医家无不关注养生，或辑先人经验，或创心法要诀，或撰养生精要，护佑中华民族繁衍生息。2021年5月，习近平总书记在全球健康峰会上发表题为《携手共建人类卫生健康共同体》的重要讲话，首次提出打造人类卫生健康共同体。中医学作为中华文明的瑰宝，其中凝聚着中华古人智慧的中医养生典籍也应当为全人类健康福祉服务。为此，我们精选《养老奉亲书》《三元参赞延寿书》《养性延命录》《饮膳正要》等经典养生古籍并译为英文，是为"中医养生经典译丛"，以飨读者。

《养老奉亲书》，宋代陈直撰，包括饮食调治、形证脉候、医药扶持、性气好嗜、宴处起居、食治老人诸疾方等内容，主要论述老年保健、四时摄养措施、疾病预防理论及治疗方法，主张老人有病，先食疗之，未愈则命药疗之，饮食宜温热熟饮、忌粘硬生冷，药饵宜用扶持之法，对老年养生具有指导意义。

《三元参赞延寿书》，元代李鹏飞撰，将人之寿命分为天元、地元、人元。"天元之寿"为"精神不耗者得之"，讨论人欲生殖，提出欲不可绝、欲不可早、欲不可纵、欲不可强、欲有所忌、欲有所避等主张；"地元之寿"为"起居有常者得之"，讨论情

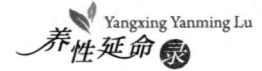

绪与起居，包括调情绪、慎起居、顺天时等；"人元之寿"为"饮食有度者得之"，讨论健康饮食，提出许多饮食养生方法。

《养性延命录》，南北朝陶弘景撰，辑录上自炎黄、下至魏晋的养生理论与方法，分上、下两卷，包括《教诫篇》《食诫篇》《杂诫忌禳害祈善篇》《服气疗病篇》《导引按摩篇》《御女损益篇》六篇，分别讲述养生理论、饮食宜忌、日常起居、行气之术、导引按摩和房中术，是道教史上对养生术的一次大总结，反映了道教学者对益寿延年的重视。

《饮膳正要》，元代忽思慧撰，是一部营养学专著，共三卷：卷一是诸般禁忌、聚珍异馔；卷二是诸般汤煎、食疗诸病及食物相反中毒等；卷三是米谷品、兽品、禽品、鱼品、果菜品和料物等。内容主要阐述各种饮馔的性味与滋补作用，还包括医疗卫生，历代名医的验方、秘方和具有蒙古族饮食特点的各种肉、乳食品，为我国现存最早的饮食卫生和食疗专书，对研究中医药，尤其是蒙古医药科技史具有重要的意义。

译者团队选取四部典籍的权威版本为蓝本，并参照多个通行本进行校勘，依据世界卫生组织、世界中医药学会联合会等颁布的标准翻译基本名词术语，力争最大限度理解和再现典籍原文内容，为中医海外从业者和研究者开展中医理论溯源和传承创新提供了研究基础。

由于译者水平有限，加之时间紧张，错讹之处敬请读者批评指正。

译者

2023 年 3 月

# 翻译说明

1. 本次所译的《养性延命录》，以钱超尘教授主编的《中华养生经典》为汉语底本，并参考了多个校注版本。

2. 典籍名称采用汉语拼音拼写，以词为拼写单位音译，括号中附以英语翻译。例如《养生要集》译为 *Yangsheng Yaoji*（*Collection of Important Health Preservation Methods*）。

3. 本书涉及少量度量单位，采用音译方法翻译，括号中附以英语翻译。例如"里"译为 Li（half a kilometer）。

4. 本书原文中有注解内容，注解与正文内容重复的不翻译。

5. 原书少量内容涉及鬼神等封建迷信，如"人为阴善，鬼神报之"，为保持经典原貌，未擅改动，供读者辨别查阅。

# Translation Specifications

1. The translation of *Yangxing Yanming Lu*（*Records on Health Preservation and Longevity*）takes its Chinese copy from *Zhonghua Yangsheng Jingdian* （*Classics on Chinese Health Preservation*）, Qian Chaochen as the editor-in-chief, with reference to other annotated editions.

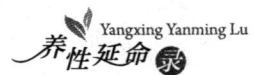

2. Names of ancient books are transliterated from Chinese characters into Pinyin according to their meanings, with their English version in brackets. For instance,《养生要集》is translated into *Yangsheng Yaoji* (*Collection of Important Health Preservation Methods*）.

3. There are a few units of measurement in the book, which are transliterated into Pinyin, with their English version in brackets. For instance, "里" is translated into Li （half a kilometer）.

4. There are annotations in the book, which are not translated when they are repetitive with the original text.

5. Some contents in this book are likely to be considered superstitious. To retain and present the original text honestly, this book made no revision of these contents and the readers are supposed to differentiate them.

本书为山东中医药大学英语专业建设成果，山东中医药大学"中医话语特征与中医翻译"青年科研创新团队成果。

# 序

## Preface

　　夫禀气含灵，唯人为贵。人所贵者，盖贵为生。生者神之本，形者神之具。神大用则竭，形大劳则毙。若能游心虚静，息虑无为，服元气于子后，时导引于闲室，摄养无亏，兼饵良药，则百年耆寿，是常分也。如恣意以耽声色，役智而图富贵，得丧恒切于怀，躁挠未能自遣，不拘礼度，饮食无节，如斯之流，宁免夭伤之患也。

Among the creatures that are endowed with the spirit of heaven and earth, human is the most precious. The most precious thing of human is life. Life is the foundation of spiritual activities, and body is the carrier of spirit. Excessive mental consumption leads to exhaustion, and immoderate physical exertion contributes to death. If people can concentrate on the emptiness and tranquility, stop worrying, let things take their own course, take original Qi after 11 O'clock in the evening, conduct in a quiet room, take good maintenance to prevent the loss of vitality, and take effective prescriptions at the same time, it should be normal to live to be a hundred years old. If people indulge in sensual and sexual behaviors,

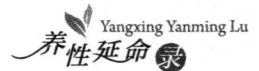

rack brains to seek wealth, worry about gain and loss, and can't adjust themselves, obey etiquette, or enjoy a good diet, can people like this still be free from the scourge of premature death and injury?

余因止观微暇，聊复披览《养生要集》。其集乃钱彦、张湛、道林之徒，翟平、黄山之辈，咸是好事英奇，志在宝育，或鸠集仙经、真人寿考之规，或得采彭铿、老君长龄之术。上自农黄以来，下及魏晋之际，但有益于养生及招损于后患，诸本先皆记录。今略取要法，删弃繁芜，类聚篇题，分为上下两卷，卷有三篇，号为《养性延命录》，拟补助于有缘，冀凭缘以济物耳。

I have some free time during my maintenance and read *Yangsheng Yaoji*（*Collection of Important Health Preservation Methods*）edited by Qian Yan, Zhang Zhan, Dao Lin, Zhai Ping, Huang Shan, etc. All of them love health preservation, possess extraordinary intelligence and indulge themselves in maintaining essence and Qi. They collect classics and warnings about longevity of immortals, and adopt the methods of Peng Keng and Lao Tzu to prolong their longevity. From Shennong and Yellow Emperor to the Wei and Jin Dynasties, things either beneficial or harmful to health preservation have been recorded in various classics. Now, I excerpt the main methods, delete the redundant content, classify and entitle them and name the book *Yangxing Yanming Lu*（*Records on Health Preservation and Longevity*）, which is divided into two volumes, three chapters for each volume. I hope this book can help people preserve health and prolong their life.

# 目 录

## Contents

# 教诫篇第一

## Chapter 1   Sermons from Ancient Classics

《神农经》曰：食谷者，智慧聪明。食石者，肥泽不老（谓炼五石也）。食芝者，延年不死。食元气者，地不能埋，天不能杀。是故食药者，与天地相弊，日月并列。

*Shennong Jing*（*Shennong's Classic of Materia Medica*）says: People who eat grain are wise and intelligent, people who take mineral medicine are lustrous and youthful, people who eat Lucid Ganoderma （Lingzhi, *Ganoderma Lucidum* seu Japonicum）can have their life prolonged, and people who breathe in original Qi can live without the negative influence of the earth and heaven. Therefore, people who take elixirs can live as long as the sun and the moon.

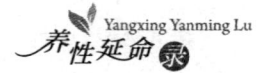

《老君道经》曰：谷神不死（河上公曰：谷，养也。能养神不死。神为五脏之神，肝藏魂，肺藏魄，心藏神，肾藏精，脾藏志。五藏尽伤，则五神去），是谓玄牝（言不死之道，在于玄牝。玄，天也，天于人为鼻；牝，地也，地于人为口。天食人以五气，从鼻入，藏于心。五气清微，为精神、聪明、音声、五性。其鬼曰魂，魂者，雄也。出入人鼻，与天通，故鼻为玄也。地食人以五味，从口入，藏于胃。五味浊滞，为形骸、骨肉、血脉、六情。其鬼曰魄，魄者，雌也。出入于口，与地通，故口为牝也）。玄牝之门，是谓天地根（根，元也。言鼻口之门，乃是天地之元气所从往来也）。绵绵若存（鼻口呼吸喘息，当绵绵微妙，若可存，复若无有也），用之不勤（用气当宽舒，不当急疾勤劳）。

*Laojun Daojing*（*Tao Ching*）says: People can have life prolonged if they nourish their spirit. And this depends on Xuan Pin（heaven and earth）. The gates of Xuan Pin, i.e. nose and mouth, serve to communicate with the heaven and earth. People should breathe gently rather than violently.

《老君德经》曰：出生（谓情欲出于五内，魂定魄静，故生也）入死（谓情欲入于胸臆，精散神惑，故死也）。生之徒十有三，死之徒十有三（言生死之类各十有三，谓之九窍四关也。其生也，目不妄视，耳不妄听，鼻不妄嗅，口不妄言，手不妄持，足不妄行，精不妄施。其死也，反是）。人之生，动之死地亦十有三（人欲求生，动作反之，十三之死地也）。夫何故？以其求生之厚也（所以动之死地者，以其求生活之太厚也。远道反天，妄行失纪）。盖闻善摄生者，陆行不遇兕虎，入军不被甲兵。兕无所投其角，虎无所措其爪，兵无所容其刃。夫何故？以其无死地（以其不犯上十三之死地也）。

*Laojun Dejing* ( *Te Ching* ) says: People can have their life prolonged without desire while people can shorten their span of life with it. There are 13 ways for people to prolong life or cause death respectively, and people going from birth to death are also due to 13 ways. Why? Because they pursue too much from life. It is said that those who know health preservation won't be attacked by rhinos or tigers when walking, or wounded by weapons in battlefields. Rhinos have nowhere to thrust their horns, tigers have nowhere to swing their paws, and weapons have nowhere to shove their edges. Why? Because they do not have Achilles' heel.

《庄子·养生篇》曰：吾生也有涯（向秀曰：生之所禀，各有极也），而智也无涯（嵇康曰：夫不虑而欲，性之动也；识而发感，智之用也。性动者，遇物而当足，则无余智；从感而求，倦而不已。故世之可患，恒在于智困，不在性动也）。以有涯随无涯，殆已（郭

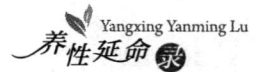
象曰：以有根之性，寻无趣之智，安得而不困哉）。已而为智者，殆而已矣（向秀曰：已困于智矣，又为智以攻之者，又殆矣）。

*Zhuangzi Yangsheng Pian* (*Health Preservation of Chuang Tzu*) says: Life is limited while knowledge is not. Thus, it is unwise to pursue unlimited desire with limited life, and it is more dangerous to pursue those you know you can't do.

《庄子》曰：达生之情者，不务生之所无以为（向秀曰：生之所无以为者，性表之事也。张湛曰：生理自全，为分外所为，此是以有涯随无涯也）。达命之情者，不务智之所无奈何（向秀曰：命尽而死者是。张湛曰：秉生顺之理，穷所禀之分，岂智所奈何）。

*Zhuangzi* (*Chuang Tzu*) says: Those who really know life do not pursue what cannot get from life; those who really know fate do not pursue what cannot change from fate.

《列子》曰：少不勤行，壮不竞时，长而安贫，老而寡欲，闲心劳形，养生之方也。

*Liezi* (*Lie Zi*) says: Do not overwork when young, do not work overtime in the prime of life, be content with poverty when old, and reduce desires to tranquilize mind and body when senile. This is the way of health preservation.

《列子》曰：一体之盈虚消息，皆通于天地，应于万类（张湛曰：人与阴阳通气）。和之于始，和之于终，静神灭想，生之道也（始终和则神志不散）。

*Liezi*（*Lie Zi*）says: The rise and fall of the body are closely connected with heaven and earth, corresponding to all things in the world. Harmonizing Yin and Yang, maintaining a peaceful mind and eliminating all desires are the ways of health preservation.

《混元妙真经》曰：人常失道，非道失人；人常去生，非生去人。故养生者，慎勿失道；为道者，慎勿失生。使道与生相守，生与道相保。

*Hunyuan Miaozhen Jing*（*Scripture of Lao Tsu*）says: People often violate the way of heaven rather than the other way around; people often abandon their life rather than the other way around. Therefore, people who know health preservation should not violate the way of heaven; people who practice Dao should not abandon their lives. In this way, the heaven and life can be protected and combined.

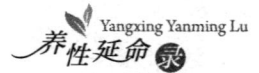
《黄老经玄示》曰：天道施化，与万物无穷；人道施化，形神消亡。转神施精，精竭故衰。形本生精，精生于神。不以精施，故能与天合德；不与神化，故能与道同式。

*Huang-Lao Jing Xuanshi（Explanation of the Yellow Emperor and Lao Tzu's Canon）* says: The way of Heaven brings about changes, making things countless and endless. However, the sexual indulgence between men and women makes people physically and mentally exhausted. Excretion of semen exhausts one's essence, resulting in exhaustion. Body is the foundation of essence, which is generated by original spirit. People can prolong life as long as heaven without frequent ejaculation, and follow the rule of Dao without deviation of spirit.

《玄示》曰：以形化者，尸解之类。神与形离，二者不俱，遂象飞鸟入海为蛤，而随季秋阴阳之气。以气化者，生可冀也；以形化者，甚可畏也。

*Xuanshi（Explanation of the Emperor Huang and Lao Tzu's Canon）* also says: Practitioners of Dao can go to the heaven with their body left. Spirit and body are separated as birds are supposed to become clams to correspond to the change of Qi of Yin and Yang in late autumn. Spirit preservation can help to prolong life while body is in danger without the coexistence of spirit.

严君平《老君指归》曰：游心于虚静，结志于微妙，委虑于无欲，归指于无为，故能达生延命，与道为久。

Yan Junping says in *Laojun Zhigui*（*Gist of Lao Tsu*）: Keep the mind in a state of emptiness and tranquility, concentrate on the subtle and mysterious things, eliminate all worries and desires, and comply to principle of non-interference. Thus life can be prolonged and people can coexist with Dao for a long time.

《大有经》曰：或疑者云：始同起于无外，终受气于阴阳，载形魄于天地，资生长于食息，而有愚有智，有强有弱，有寿有夭，天耶？人耶？解者曰：夫形生愚智，天也；强弱寿夭，人也。天道自然，人道自己。始而胎气充实，生而乳食有余，长而滋味不足，壮而声色有节者，强而寿；始而胎气虚耗，生而乳食不足，长而滋味有余，壮而声色自放者，弱而夭。生长全足，加之导养，年未可量。

*Dayou Jing*（*Classic of Dayou Palace*）says: Some people ask suspiciously that all people originated from chance at first, and finally were dominated by the Qi of Yin and Yang. Their body and spirit exist between heaven and earth and all lived by eating and

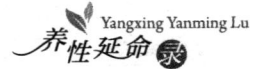

breathing. However, they are either ignorant or intelligent, strong or weak, longevous or ephemeral. Is this caused by heaven? Or human beings? The wise man says: Ignorance or intelligence is decided by heaven, while body constitution and longevity are determined by human. The law of heaven cannot be changed while life can be prolonged by postnatal effort. If one develops fully at the beginning of pregnancy, has enough milk to suckle after his birth, and doesn't overindulge in delicious food when growing up or immerse in sensual and sexual pleasure in the prime of life, he can be strong and longevous, but doing the opposite makes him weak and ephemeral. If one develops fully, maintains properly and conducts frequently, he is bound to live long.

《道机》曰：人生而命有长短者，非自然也。皆由将身不谨，饮食过差，淫泆无度，忤逆阴阳，魂神不守，精竭命衰，百病萌生，故不终其寿。

*Daoji*（*Secret of Tao*）says: People's life expectancy is either long or short, which is not determined by heaven. On the contrary, the improper maintenance of the body, poor diet, overindulgence in sex, and violence of Yin and Yang lead to the disturbance of spirit and even various diseases. Thus, they can't live a long life.

《河图帝视萌》曰：侮天时者凶，顺天时者吉。春夏乐山高处，秋冬居卑深藏，吉利多福，寿考无穷。

*Hetu Dishi Meng*（*Yellow Emperor's Outing*）says: People who despise heaven and earth are ominous, while those who conform to the nature are auspicious. In spring and summer, people should climb mountains and live in high places, while in autumn and winter, people should live in low places and hide themselves. In this way, people will have good luck and long life.

《洛书宝予命》曰：古人治病之方，和以醴泉，润以元气，药不辛不苦，甘甜多味，常能服之，津流五脏，系在心肺，终身无患。

*Luoshu Baoyuming*（*Classic for Health Preservation*）says: When the ancient people treat diseases, they boil medicine with sweet spring water and moisten with original Qi. Such medicine is not spicy or bitter, but sweet instead. Taking this medicine frequently makes the body fluid flow into the five zang–organs, and regulate the heart and lung, so people do not suffer from diseases for their whole life.

《孔子家语》曰：食肉者，勇敢而悍（虎狼之类）；食气者，

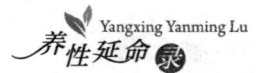
神明而寿（仙人、灵龟是也）；食谷者，智慧而夭（人也）；不食者，不死而神（直任喘息而无思虑）。

*Kongzi Jiayu*（*The Family Sayings of Confucius*）says: Those who mainly eat meat tend to be brave and valiant（such as tigers and wolves）; those who take Qi tend to be energetic and longevous（such as immortals and turtles）; those who eat grain are intelligent but ephemeral（such as humans）; those who seldom eat but frequently practice can live long and become immortals（such as practitioners who conduct by breath without anxiety）.

《传》曰：杂食者，百病妖邪所钟。所食愈少，心愈开，年愈益；所食愈多，心愈塞，年愈损焉。

*Zhuan*（*Records of Immortals*）says: People who eat disorderly are prone to diseases. The less people eat and the more open-minded they are, the longer they live; the more people eat and the more narrow-minded they are, the shorter they live.

太史公司马谈曰：夫神者，生之本；形者，生之具也。神大用则竭，形大劳则毙。神形早衰，欲与天地长久，非所闻也。故人所以生者，神也；神之所托者，形也。神形离别则死，死者不可复生，离者不可复返，故乃圣人重之。夫养生之道，有都领大归，未能具其会者，但思每与俗反，则暗践胜辙，获过半之功矣。有心之徒，可不察欤？

Sima Tan says: Spirit is the foundation of life while body is the carrier of life. Excessive spirit consumption leads to exhaustion and overwork to death. It is unheard-of to live a long life with premature mental and physical exhaustion. Therefore, people can live by virtue of spirit, which in turn relies on the body. If the spirit is separated from the body, people will die, and the detached spirit and body cannot be combined. Therefore, the saints attach great importance to the maintenance of body and spirit. There is a general outline to maintain health. Even if you can't fully understand it, as long as your behavior is contrary to secular habits, it will coincide with the way to maintain health and thus obtain at least half success. Can anyone who wants to maintain health not care about this?

《小有经》曰：少思、少念、少欲、少事、少语、少笑、少愁、少乐、少喜、少怒、少好、少恶，行此十二少，乃养生之都契也。多思则神怠，多念则志散，多欲则损智，多事则形疲，多语则气争，多笑则伤藏，多愁则心慑，多乐则意溢，多喜则忘错昏乱，多怒则百脉不定，多好则专迷不治，多恶则焦煎无欢。此十二多不除，丧生之本也。无多者，几乎真人。大计奢懒者寿，悭勤者夭，

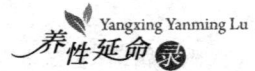

放散劬劳之异也。田夫寿，膏粱夭，嗜欲多少之验也。处士少疾，游子多患，事务繁简之殊也。故俗人竞利，道士罕营。

*Xiaoyou Jing*（*Classic of Xiaoyou Palace*）says: The twelve lesses—less thinking, delusion, desire, work, speech, laughter, sorrow, leisure, ecstasy, anger, indulgence and disgust—are the general principles of health preservation. Too much thinking weakens spirit, too much delusion scatters emotion, too much desire damages sanity, too much work exhausts body, too much speech presses breath, too much laughter injures the organs, too much sorrow leads to fear, too much leisure dissipates will, too much ecstasy disturbs spirit, too much anger blocks meridians, too much indulgence makes one ignore duties, and too much disgust yields suffering. These are the root causes of the damage to life. Get rid of these excessive things, and hence humans will become immortal beings. Generally speaking, people who are comfortable and idle can live a longer life while those who are frugal and overtired live shorter. This difference is caused by relaxation and exhaustion. Farmers live a longer life, while dignitaries live shorter. This is caused by different hobbies and desires. People who live stably are less vulnerable to diseases than those wandering. This is caused by different indulgence in affairs. Therefore, people in the secular world strive for fame and fortune, while those who preserve health do not.

胡昭曰：目不欲视不正之色，耳不欲听丑秽之言，鼻不欲向膻腥之气，口不欲尝毒辣之味，心不欲谋欺诈之事，此辱神损寿。又居常而叹息，晨夜而吟啸，干正来邪也。夫常人不得无欲，又复不得无事，但当和心少念，静身损虑，先去乱神犯性之事，此则啬神之一术也。

Hu Zhao says: People should not look at the wicked color, listen to the filthy speech, smell the fishy odor, taste the spicy flavor or plan the fraud, because these acts are blasphemous and will reduce life expectancy. In addition, moaning and sighing all day, shouting and howling in the morning and dusk, will interfere with healthy Qi and invite filth. Ordinary people cannot live without desire or idle away their time, so they should harmonize mind and spirit, reduce delusions and stabilize their thinking. Above all, they should get rid of the acts that disturb their mind, and this is a method of health preservation through cherishing the spirit.

《黄庭经》曰：玉池清水灌灵根，审能修之可长存。名曰饮食自然。自然者，则是华池。华池者，口中唾也。呼吸如法，咽之则不饥也。

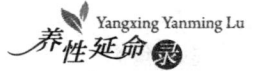
*Huangting Jing*（*Huangting Classic*）says: Swallowing saliva in your mouth can nourish the body. If people can seriously practice this method, they can live a long life. If they breathe properly and often swallow saliva, they won't feel hungry.

《老君尹氏内解》曰：唾者，漱为醴泉，聚为玉浆，流为华池，散为精汋，降为甘露。故口为华池，中有醴泉，漱而咽之，溉藏润身，流利百脉，化养万神，肢节毛发宗之而生也。

*Laojun Yinshi Neijie*（*Yin's Explanation of Lao Tsu*）says: There is sweet saliva in the mouth. Saliva can be rinsed in the mouth like spring, gathered like nectar, circulated like pond, scattered like essence and descended like sweet dew. Gargling and swallowing saliva can help to moisten the five zang-organs, and then saliva infuses meridians and promotes various functions of the body. And hence body hair grows.

《中经》曰：静者寿，躁者夭。静而不能养减寿，躁而能养延年。然静易御，躁难持，尽顺养之宜者，则静亦可养，躁亦可养。

*Zhongjing*（*Middle Classic*）says: Quiet people live long while restless people live short. Quiet people who don't know health preservation also reduce life expectancy and restless people who know it can also prolong life. However, quietness is easy to handle but restlessness isn't. If people, either quiet or restless, follow the law of health preservation, they can both maintain health.

韩融元长曰：酒者，五谷之华，味之至也，亦能损人。然美物难将而易过，养性所宜慎之。

Han Rong says: Liquor is the essence of five cereals and the best flavor in the diet, but it can also harm people. However, it is always difficult for people to control desire for liquor and easy to indulge in it, and thus people who preserve health should be cautious.

邵仲堪曰：五谷充肌体而不能益寿，百药疗疾延年而不能甘口。充肌甘口者，俗人之所珍。苦口延年者，道士之所宝。

Shao Zhongkan says: Five cereals can replenish and nourish the body but cannot prolong life, while drugs can cure diseases and prolong life but taste bitter. Those sweet and nourishing cereals are cherished by average people while those bitter and macrobiotic drugs are valued by those who know health preservation.

《素问》曰：黄帝问岐伯曰：余闻上古之人，春秋皆百岁而动作不衰（谓血气犹盛也）；今时之人，年所始半百动作皆衰者，

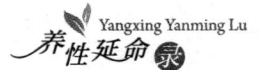

时世异耶？将人之失耶？岐伯曰：上古之人，其知道者，法则阴阳，和于术数（房中交接之法），饮食有节，起居有度，不妄动作，故能形与神俱，尽终其天命，寿过百岁；今时之人则不然，以酒为浆，以妄为常，醉以入房，以欲竭其精，以好散其真，不知持满，不时御神，务快其心，逆于阴阳，治生起居无节无度，故半百而衰也。

Suwen（Plain Questions）says: Yellow Emperor asked Master Qibo: "I've heard that people in ancient times could live about one hundred years without any decline in action. But people today begin to be doddery even at the age of fifty. Is it due to the variation of times or the violation of the way to preserve health?" Qibo answered: "People in ancient times, who knew the way to preserve health, could follow the rules of Yin and Yang and sexual regimen. They were moderate in eating and drinking, regular in working and resting, and could avoid any overstrain. That is why they could maintain a desirable harmony between the spirit and the body, enjoy good health and a long life. People today behave just oppositely. They drink liquor as thin rice gruel, regard indulgence as normal, and seek sexual pleasure after drinking. Therefore, their essence is exhausted and genuine Qi is dissipated. They seldom keep an exuberance of essence and don't accommodate spirit regularly, but instead do whatever they like while violating the law of life enjoyment and live an irregular life. That's why they are aging at the age of fifty."

《老子》曰：人生大期，百年为限，节护之者，可至千岁。如膏之用，小炷与大耳。众人大言而我小语，众人多烦而我少记，众人悖暴而我不怒，不以人事累意，不修君臣之义，淡然无为，神气自满，以为不死之药，天下莫我知也。无谓幽冥，天和人情，无谓暗昧，神见人形。心言小语，鬼闻人声；犯禁满干，地收人形。人为阳善，正人报之；人为阴善，鬼神报之。人为阳恶，正人治之；人为阴恶，鬼神治之。故天不欺人依以影，地不欺人依以响。

*Laozi*（*Lao Tzu*）says: The life span of a person is about a hundred years. Those who can control and maintain their life can live to a thousand years. Just like lighting an oil lamp, the burning time varies with the size of the wick. People speak loudly while I whisper softly, people worry much while I don't think about those trivial things, people are frightened and furious while I'm not angry. I don't encumber my mind with all kinds of things, including etiquette with the monarch, or pursue fame and fortune, I cultivate my mind and I am thus energetic. This is the real medicine for longevity, and I know it well. There is no place too remote to reach because the heaven

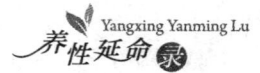

knows; there is no place too dim to identify because the divinity knows. The ghosts and divinities can hear people's voice even if it is a whisper. If a man breaks the taboo a thousand times, he will die. If a man does good works in public, benevolent people will repay him; if a man does good deeds in secret, ghosts and divinities will repay him. If a man does evil things openly, benevolent people will punish him; if a man does evil things secretly, ghosts and divinities will punish him. Therefore, heaven does not bully people, just like shadow goes together with shape; the earth does not bully people, just like sound goes together with explosion.

老君曰：人修善积德而遇其凶祸者，受先人之余殃也；犯禁为恶而遇其福者，蒙先人之余福也。

Lao Tzu says: People do good deeds but still encounter dangerous disasters, because they are implicated by the sins of their ancestors; people violate taboos and commit evils but still encounter blessings, because they are sheltered by the blessings of their ancestors.

《名医叙病论》曰：世人不终耆寿，咸多夭殁者，皆由不自爱惜，忿争尽意，邀名射利，聚毒攻神，内伤骨体，外乏筋肉，血气将无，经脉便壅，内里空疏，惟招众疾，正气日衰，邪气日盛矣。不异举沧波以注爝火，颓华岳而断涓流，语其易也，甚于兹矣。

*Mingyi Xubing Lun*（*Famous Doctor's Discussion on Diseases*）says: The reason why people don't live as long as they deserve is that they don't care about their body. They worry and anger at will, pursue fame and fortune, invite evil thoughts and invade original spirit, which injures bones internally, damages muscles externally, exhausts blood and Qi, blocks meridians and thus they invite various diseases. In this way, healthy Qi declines every day and pathogenic Qi grows stronger accordingly. It's the same as using the water of the sea to extinguish candles and push down Huashan （a big mountain）to cut off streams. This metaphor is not meant to terrify, but the actual situation is much more terrible.

彭祖曰：道不在烦，但能不思衣，不思食，不思声，不思色，不思胜，不思负，不思失，不思得，不思荣，不思辱，心不劳，形不极，常导引、纳气、胎息尔，可得千岁，欲长生无限者，当服上药。

Peng Zu says: The key to health preservation does not lie in diversity of methods. As long as they don't pursue luxuriant food and clothing, indulge in sensual and sexual pleasure, fuss about things like victory or defeat, gain or loss, honor or disgrace, or overstrain the body

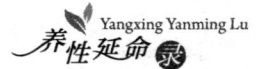

and mind, but instead oftentimes conduct and absorb Qi deeply, they can live to a thousand years old. If people want to live forever, they must take the best medicine for health preservation.

仲长统曰：荡六情五性，有心而不以之思，有口而不以之言，有体而不以之安。安之而能迁，乐之而不爱。以之图之，不知日之益也，不知物之易也，彭祖、老聃庶几，不然，彼何为与人者同类，而与人者异寿？

Zhong Changtong says: People should cast off the six emotions and five temperaments; don't think too much, don't talk much, and don't seek too much physical comfort. They should often work even if there is a comfortable life; they may like something but should not overindulge. They should forget the passage of time and the changes of things following these principles. Peng Zu and Lao Tzu may have done it. Otherwise, why are they the same as ordinary people, but their life expectancy is very different from them?

陈纪元方曰：百病横夭，多由饮食。饮食之患，过于声色。声色可绝之逾年，饮食不可废之一日。为益亦多，为患亦切（多则切伤，少则增益）。

Chen Ji says: Various diseases are rampant mostly due to

improper diet. The harm of improper diet exceeds that of sensual and sexual pleasure. People can abstain from sensual and sexual pleasure all year long, but cannot live for a single day without food and drink. Diet has many benefits to the human body, but the harm it brings to people is also serious （excessive diet will do great harm while and less diet will be beneficial to the body）.

张湛云：凡贵权势者，虽不中邪，精神内伤，身必死亡（非妖祸外侵，直由冰炭内煎，则自崩伤中呕血）。始富后贫，虽不中邪，皮焦筋出，委痹为挛（贫富之于人，利害犹于权势，故病疹损于形骸）。动胜寒，静胜热，能动能静，所以长生。精气清净，乃与道合。

Zhang Zhan says: Those moguls who lose power will die due to internal mental damage, even if they are not invaded by pathogenic Qi （The damage is not caused by invasion from the outside, but by mental suffering due to emotional fluctuation, which leads to damage to internal organs or even hematemesis）. Those rich people who come down in the world will suffer withered skin, exposed tendons, limb weakness and spasm （The damage of wealth to people is the same as power, so diseases occur and damage the body）. Movement can drive out cold while quietness can overcome heat, and thus movement and

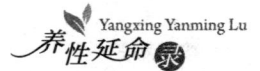

quietness make people live long. Only when the spirit is pure and quiet can it comply with Dao.

《庄子》曰：真人其寝不梦。

*Zhuangzi（Chuang Tzu）* says: Those immortals do not dream while sleep.

《慎子》云：昼无事者夜不梦。

*Shenzi（Shen Zi）* says: People won't dream at night if nothing bothers during the day.

张道人年百数十，甚翘壮也，云：养性之道，莫久行、久坐、久卧、久听，莫强食饮，莫大醉，莫大愁忧，莫大哀思，此所谓能中和。能中和者，必久寿也。

Taoist Zhang is over a hundred years old and he is still very strong. He says: Health preservation requires that people should not walk, sit, lie, or listen overtime. Don't be crapulent, drunk, worry or sad, and this is what we call neutralization. Those who can balance themselves are bound to live long.

《仙经》曰：我命在我不在于天，但愚人不能知此道为生命之要。所以致百病风邪者，皆由恣意极情，不知自惜，故虚损生也。譬如枯朽之木，遇风即折；将崩之岸，值水先颓。今若不能服药，但知爱精节情，亦得一二百年寿也。

*Xianjing*（*Immortal Classic*）says: My life is dominated by myself instead of heaven, but fools don't know that health preservation is the core of life. Various diseases are caused by unscrupulous behaviors and ignorance of self-care, which damage their lives. Withered and decayed trees break easily when they encounter the wind; the bank that is about to collapse crumbles first when facing water. Now, even if people don't take the elixir for health preservation, they can still live to one or two hundred years old as long as they preserve essence and control desire.

张湛《养生集叙》曰：养生大要：一曰啬神，二曰爱气，三曰养形，四曰导引，五曰言语，六曰饮食，七曰房室，八曰反俗，九曰医药，十曰禁忌。过此以往，义可略焉。

Zhang Zhan says in *Yangsheng Jixu*（*Collection of Health Preservation*）: The key points of health preservation are: first, save the spirit; second, cherish Qi; third, maintain the body; fourth, conduct Qi; fifth, be cautious in speech; sixth, control diet; seventh, avoid sexual indulgence; eighth, deviate from the secular world;

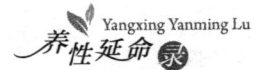

ninth, understand medicine; tenth, abide by taboos. These are the most important principles for health preservation.

青牛道士言：人不欲使乐，乐人不寿，但当莫强为力所不任，举重引强，掘地苦作，倦而不息，以致筋骨疲竭耳。然劳苦胜于逸乐也。能从朝至暮常有所为，使之不息乃快，但觉极当息，息复为之。此与导引无异也。夫流水不腐，户枢不朽者，以其劳动数故也。饱食不用坐与卧，欲得行步，务作以散之。不尔，使人得积聚不消之疾，及手足痹蹶，面目黧皱，必损年寿也。

Taoist Feng Heng, also known as black ox Taoist, says: People can't be too comfortable, and a cozy life makes people not live long. People should not force themselves to do things that they can't do, such as lifting heavy objects, pulling a strong bow, digging earth, and other heavy work. If they are tired and don't rest, they will be exhausted. However, proper labor is better than idling. They can always do proper things from morning to night, which is beneficial to health. Rest when they feel tired and resume their work after that. This has the same effect as conduction exercise. The reason why a rolling stone gathers no moss is that it moves about frequently. Thus, people should not sit or lie down after diet, but instead, they should take a walk or labor to digest food. Otherwise, they are prone to diseases caused by retention of food, paralysis and numbness of hands and feet, inconvenient walking and dark complexion, which will certainly damage their life.

皇甫隆问青牛道士（青牛道士姓封，字君达，其养性法则可施用）。大略云：体欲常劳，食欲常少，劳无过极，少无过虚。去肥浓，节咸酸，减思虑，损喜怒，除驰逐，慎房室。武帝行之有效。

Huangfu Long asks black ox Taoist（His name is Feng Junda and his methods work）about health preservation. He answers: People should work frequently and eat less, and they should work but not overwork, eat less but not starve to hunger. People should abstain from the fat, sweet and greasy diet, control the sour and salty taste, reduce thinking and worry, give up the capricious mood, stop hunting and chasing activities, and control sexual affairs. Emperor Wu of Han dynasty followed these rules and they worked.

彭祖曰：人受气，虽不知方术，但养之得理，常寿一百二十岁。不得此者，皆伤之也。少复晓道，可得二百四十岁。复微加药物，可得四百八十岁（嵇康亦云：道养得理，上可寿千岁，下可寿百岁）。

Peng Zu says: People are nurtured by the Qi of nature. Even if

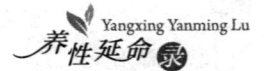

they don't know medicine, divination or similar arts, they can often live to 120 years old as long as they are properly maintained. Those who fail to meet the age are all caused by injury to body. If they follow health preservation rule from young age, they can live to 240 years old. If they take some elixirs, they can reach 480 years old （Ji Kang also says: Those who follow health preservation rules properly can reach 1000 years old or at least a hundred）.

彭祖曰：养寿之法，但莫伤之而已。夫冬温夏凉，不失四时之和，所以适身也。重衣厚褥，体不堪苦，以致风寒之疾；厚味脯腊，醉饱厌饫，以致聚结之疾；美色妖丽，嫔妾盈房，以致虚损之祸；淫声哀音，怡心悦耳，以致荒耽之惑；驰骋游观，弋猎原野，以致发狂之失；谋得战胜，兼弱取乱，以致骄逸之败。盖圣贤或失其理也。然养生之具，譬犹水火，不可失适，反为害耳。

Peng Zu says: To maintain health and longevity, people shouldn't hurt their body. Keep warm in winter, keep cool in summer, and harmonize the body based on the changes of the four seasons, and these are proper methods for human conditions. If they wear too much or pad too thick in bed, the body suffers, which weakens the ability to resist the wind and cold and thus disease arises. If they take too much fat, sweet and greasy food and drink too much, disease occurs due to retention of food. If they seek too much sexual pleasure, have too many wives and concubines, diseases appear due to overconsumption of essence and semen. If they indulge in obscene sounds and mournful music, they suffer from debauchery and confusion. If they gallop and wander, or hunt in the field frequently, they become profligate and unrestrained. If they win by trick, annex the weak and take profits from chaos, they become arrogant. Perhaps some sages have not mastered the principle of health preservation and thus have a short life. Various methods of health preservation, like using water and fire, cannot go beyond the limit, or they will become disasters.

彭祖曰：人不知道，经服药损伤，血气不足，内理空疏，髓脑不实，内已先病，故为外物所犯，风寒酒色以发之耳。若本充实，岂有病乎？

Peng Zu says: People who do not know how to maintain health take medicine directly when they are ill, which results in physical damage. When Qi and blood are deficient, the internal organs and striae are sloppy, the brain and marrow are not full, they are already sick inside the body. So, when they are invaded by external pathogens, or suffer from wind, cold or liquor, diseases will be induced. If they are

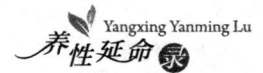

strong enough, how can they get sick?

仙人曰：罪莫大于淫，祸莫大于贪，咎莫大于谗。此三者祸之车，小则危身，大则危家。若欲延年少病者，诚勿施精，施精命夭残。勿大温消骨髓，勿大寒伤肌肉，勿咳唾失肌汁，勿卒呼惊魂魄，勿久泣神悲戚，勿恚怒神不乐，勿念内志恍惚，能行此道，可以长生。

The immortal says: There is no greater sin than promiscuity, no greater disaster than greed, and no greater fault than slander. These three things are the origins of disaster, which harm people themselves or even their family. If people want to prolong life and reduce diseases, they should be warned not to ejaculate in sexual intercourse frequently. Frequent ejaculation makes people short-lived. Do not stay in extremely hot environment, which dissolves the bone marrow; don't stay in extremely cold environment, which damages muscles; don't spit too much saliva, which makes people lose body fluid; don't shout suddenly, which disturbs the soul; don't cry for a long time, which causes depression; don't be angry, which troubles the mind; don't indulge in sex, which makes people absent-minded. If people can follow these methods, they can live a long life.

# 食诚篇第二

## Chapter 2　Food Prohibition

真人曰：虽常服药物，而不知养性之术，亦难以长生也。养性之道，不欲饱食便卧及终日久坐，皆损寿也。人欲小劳，但莫至疲及强所不能堪胜耳。人食毕，当行步踌躇，有所修为为快也。故流水不腐，户枢不蠹，以其劳动数故也。故人不要夜食，食毕但当行中庭，如数里可佳。饱食即卧生百病，不消成积聚也。食欲少而数，不欲顿多难销。常如饱中饥，饥中饱。故养性者，先饥乃食，先渴而饮。恐觉饥乃食，食必多；盛渴乃饮，饮必过。食毕当行，行毕使人以粉摩腹数百过，大益也。

The immortal says: Even if people often take tonifying medicine, it is difficult for them to live long without knowing health preservation. The key is not to lie in bed immediately after they are stuffed, nor sit for a long time all day, all of which will cut people's lifespan. Light physical labor is necessary, but it should not be too much to exhaust people or exceed the endurance limit of the body. After meals, people should take a leisurely walk because proper exercises make them happy and satisfied. The reason why a rolling stone gathers no moss is that it moves about frequently. Therefore, people should not eat much at night. If they do, it is advisable for them to take a walk in the courtyard for a few Li（half a kilometer）. Lying down immediately after being stuffed makes people suffer from all kinds of diseases due to indigestion. People should have more meals a day but less food for each. Do not eat too much at a time, which makes it difficult to digest. It is suggested to maintain a state between fullness and hunger. Therefore, people who preserve health take food before they feel hungry and drink water before they feel thirsty. That's probably because if people eat when hungry, they tend to overeat; if people drink water when thirsty, they tend to drink too much. Take a walk after meal, and then it is beneficial to have the abdomen massaged hundreds of times with talcum powder.

青牛道士言：食不欲过饱，故道士先饥而食也。饮不欲过多，故道士先渴而饮也。食毕行数百步，中益也。暮食毕，行五里许乃卧，令人除病。凡食，先欲得食热食，次食温暖食，次冷食。食热暖食讫，如无冷食者，即吃冷水一两咽，甚妙。若能恒记，即是养性之要法也。凡食，欲得先微吸取气，咽一两咽，乃食，主无病。

Black ox Taoist says: Don't eat too much, that's why Taoists always take food before hunger. Don't drink too much water, that's why Taoists drink water before thirst. It is beneficial to take hundreds of steps after meal. Walking for about 5 Li（2.5 kilometers）before sleeping at night can keep people from getting sick. In general, when eating, hot food should be taken first, then warm food, finally cold food. If there is no cold food after eating hot or warm food, swallow one or two mouthfuls of cold water instead. Bear this in mind, and people can master an important method of health preservation. People should first inhale slightly and then swallow once or twice before eating to avoid getting sick.

真人言：热食伤骨，冷食伤脏；热物灼唇，冷物痛齿。食讫踟蹰，长生。饱食勿大语。大饮则血脉闭，大醉则神散。

The immortal says: Hot food damages bones, while cold food injures the internal organs; hot food burns the lips, while cold food hurts the teeth. Walking after meal helps to prolong people's life. Do

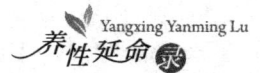

not speak aloud after eating. If people drink too much, the blood vessels will be blocked, and the spirit will be dissipated after being drunk.

春宜食辛，夏宜食酸，秋宜食苦，冬宜食咸，此皆助五脏，益血气，辟诸病。食酸咸甜苦，即不得过分食。春不食肝，夏不食心，秋不食肺，冬不食肾，四季不食脾。如能不食此五脏，尤顺天理。燕不可食，入水为蛟蛇所吞，亦不宜杀之。饱食讫即卧，成病背痛。饮酒不欲多，多即吐，吐不佳。醉卧不可当风，亦不可用扇，皆损人。

It is suitable to eat spicy food in spring, sour food in summer, bitter food in autumn, and salty food in winter. These foods can help nourish the five zang-organs, replenish blood and Qi, and avoid various diseases, but should not be overeaten. Don't eat animal's liver in spring, heart in summer, lung in autumn, kidney in winter and spleen in all seasons. If people do not eat these five zang-organs of animals, they actually comply with the way of nature. People should not eat swallows, otherwise they will be swallowed by water snakes when they fall into the water, and swallows should not be killed either. Lying in bed on a full stomach tends to cause back pain. Don't drink too much, because excessive drinking contributes to vomit which is not good to health. People should not lie down in a windy place nor use a fan when they are drunk, both of which are harmful to the body.

白蜜勿合李子同食，伤五内。醉不可强食，令人发痈疽，生疮。醉饱交接，小者令人面皯、咳嗽，不幸伤绝脏脉，损命。凡食，欲得恒温暖，宜入易消，胜于习冷。凡食，皆熟胜于生，少胜于多。饱食走马成心痴。饮水勿忽咽之，成气病及水癖。人食酪，勿食酢，变为血痰及尿血。食热食汗出，勿洗面，令人失颜色，面如虫行。食热食讫，勿以醋浆漱口，令人口臭及血齿。马汗息及马毛入食中，亦能害人。鸡、兔、犬肉，不可合食。

Don't eat white honey and plum at the same time, which injures the five zang-organs. Don't overeat after being drunk, which causes carbuncle and sore. Intercourse after drinking and eating too much causes dark complexion and cough in mild cases, and in severe cases it may hurt meridians in the five zang-organs and even damage life.

In general, it is better to eat warm, palatable and digestible food than cold food. Meanwhile, cooked food is better than raw food, and less food is better than excessive food. Riding a horse on a full stomach is prone to cause unconsciousness and delusion. Don't swallow in a hurry when drinking water, which leads to Qi-related disease or thoracic fluid retention. Don't take vinegar after eating cheese, or it causes bloody sputum and hematuria. Don't wash face immediately

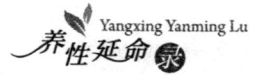

after sweating from eating hot food, or it makes people look bad and feel like insects crawling on the face. Don't rinse mouth with vinegar after eating hot food, or it causes ozostomia and tooth bleeding. If mucus from horse's nose, the horse's breath and hair mix into the food, it will do harm to people. Chicken, rabbit, and dog meat cannot be cooked and eaten together.

烂茆屋上水滴侵者脯，名曰郁脯，食之损人。久饥不得饱食，饱食成癖病。饱食夜卧失覆，多霍乱死。时病新差，勿食生鱼，成痢不止。食生鱼，勿食乳酪，变成虫。食兔肉，勿食干姜，成霍乱。人食肉，不用取上头最肥者，必众人先目之，食者变成结气及疰疬，食皆然。空腹勿食生果，令人膈上热，骨蒸，作痈疖。

The preserved meat infiltrated by the water drop of rotten thatched eaves, known as rotten preserved meat, will damage the body if eaten. Don't eat too much after being hungry for a long time, which leads to lumps. Sleeping without a quilt at night on a full stomach tends to cause death from cholera. Don't eat fresh fish right after recovering from seasonal diseases, which is prone to cause diarrhea. Don't take cheese after eating fresh fish, which is prone to cause parasites. Don't take dried ginger after eating rabbit meat, which is prone to cause cholera. Don't eat the fattest part of the meat, which must have been first noticed by everyone. Eating such meat tends to cause Qi stagnation and chronic infectious diseases. Don't eat raw fruit on an empty stomach, which is prone to cause fever on the diaphragm, steaming bone fever and carbuncle.

铜器盖食，汗出落食中，食之发疮，肉疽。触寒未解食热食，亦作刺风。饮酒热未解，勿以冷水洗面，令人面发疮。饱食勿沐发，沐发令人作头风。荞麦和猪肉食，不过三顿成热风。干脯勿置秫米瓮中，食之闭气。干脯火烧不动，出火始动，擘之筋缕相交者，食之患人或杀人。羊脾中有肉如珠子者，名羊悬筋，食之患癫痫。诸湿食之不见形影者，食之成疰，腹胀。

Covering food with bronze ware may generate steam droplets. Once they drop into food and are taken by people, sores and carbuncles may occur. If people eat hot food before recovering from wind cold, they may suffer from stabbing pain. Don't wash face with cold water before the drunk heat being dissipated, otherwise people may get sores on face. Don't wash hair on a full stomach, otherwise people may get recurrent headache. Eating buckwheat together with pork about three times can cause heat wind. Eating dried meat preserved in the husked sorghum urn leads to stagnation of Qi movement. Eating the preserved

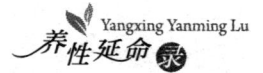
meat, which cannot swell when burned in the fire but starts to swell after being taken out, the tendons being crisscrossed if it is cut open, makes people sick or even die. Eating the bead-like meat balls in the scapula of sheep, which is called sheep hanging tendons, causes epilepsy. Eating rotten food whose true color can no longer be figured out leads to chronic diseases and abdominal distension.

暴疾后不周饮酒，膈上变热。新病差不用食生枣、羊肉、生菜，损颜色，终身不复，多致死，膈上热蒸。凡食热脂饼物，不用饮冷醋、浆水，善失声若咽。生葱白合蜜食，害人，切忌。干脯得水自动，杀人。曝肉作脯，不肯燥，勿食。羊肝勿合椒食，伤人心。胡瓜合羊肉食之，发热。多酒食肉，名曰痴脂，忧狂无恒。食良药、五谷充悦者，名曰中士，犹虑疾苦。食气，保精存神，名曰上士，与天同年。

Don't drink alcohol after contracting acute illness, otherwise it may cause fever on the diaphragm. Don't eat raw jujubes, mutton, or lettuce immediately after recovering from illness, which damages the complexion and it can't get recovered for life, and tends to lead to death or fever on the diaphragm when you eat too much. Don't drink cold vinegar or Jiangshui（a sour beverage in ancient China）when eating hot oily cakes, which is prone to make people hoarse or lose voice. Eating raw scallion and honey together is harmful and should be abstained. Eating preserved meat which fluctuate on its own after being soaked in water leads to damage. Don't eat the meat which cannot be dried after being exposed to the sun for a long time when processing preserved meat. Don't eat lamb liver with Chinese prickly ash, which hurts people's heart. Eating cucumber with mutton together makes people feverish. Gluttons for meat and wine, known as Chizhi（people who are obsessed with grease）, tend to be depressed, manic and impatient. People who take good medicine and feed on the five cereals know health preservation, though they are still worried about the pain of disease. People who take Qi and preserve the essence and the spirit can prolong life as long as heaven.

# 杂诫忌禳害祈善篇第三

## Chapter 3　Taboos, Disasters and Blessings

久视伤血，久卧伤气，久立伤骨，久行伤筋，久坐伤肉。远思强健伤人，忧恚悲哀伤人，喜乐过差伤人，忿怒不解伤人，汲汲所愿伤人，戚戚所患伤人，寒暖失节伤人，阴阳不交伤人。凡交，须依导引诸术。若能避众伤之事，而复晓阴阳之术，则是不死之道。大乐气飞扬，大愁气不通。用精令人气力乏，多视令人目盲，多唾令人心烦，贪美食令人泄痢。

Protracted seeing damages blood, protracted lying damages Qi, protracted standing damages bones, protracted walking damages tendons, and protracted sitting damages muscles. Excessive thought and overstrain hurts people, so does melancholy, sorrow, excessive joy and constant anger. The eager to pursue the realization of desire hurts people, so does endless sorrow for the suffering and unbalanced cold and hot, and the same is true if there is no sexual intercourse between men and women. All sexual intercourse between men and women should be done in accordance with conduction methods. If people can avoid all kinds of damages and master the art of sexual intercourse, it is the way towards immortality. Excessive joy scatters Qi while excessive sorrow blocks Qi. Consuming essence and Qi makes people tired, seeing too much makes people blind, spitting too much makes people distracted, and eating too much makes people suffer from diarrhea.

俗人但知贪于五味，不知有元气可饮。圣人知五味之毒焉，故不贪，知元气可服，故闭口不言，精气自应也。唾不咽则海不润，海不润则津液乏，是以服元气、饮醴泉，乃延年之本也。

Ordinary people are greedy for five flavors, but they don't know there is original Qi to consume. The sages know the harm of five flavors, so they are not greedy. They know there is original Qi, so they shut up and the essence will naturally correspond. If people don't swallow saliva oftentimes, the sea of Qi can't be moistened, and the body fluid is insufficient consequently. Therefore, it can be seen that taking original Qi and swallowing saliva is the foundation of prolonging life.

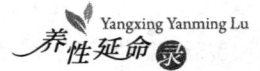

沐浴无常不吉，夫妇同浴不吉。新沐浴及醉饱，远行归还大疲倦，并不可行房室之事，生病，切慎之。丈夫勿头北向卧，令人神不安，多愁忘。勿跂井，今古大忌。若见十步地墙，勿顺墙坐卧，被风吹发癫痫疾。勿怒目久视日月，使目睛失明。

It's unlucky not to bath regularly. It's unlucky for couples to bathe together. People can't have sex right after taking a bath, being drunk or full, or tired after a long trip, otherwise they are vulnerable to diseases. A husband should not sleep with his head pointing to the north, otherwise it will make people nervous, worried and forgetful. Don't sit by the well, which is a big taboo since ancient times. If people see a ten-meter low wall, don't sit and lie down along the wall to avoid possible epilepsy caused by the pathogenic wind. Don't stare at the sun and moon for a long time, which makes the eyes blind.

凡大汗勿脱衣，不慎多患偏风，半身不遂。新沐浴讫不得露头当风，不幸得大风刺风疾。触寒来勿面临火上，成痫，起风眩头痛。勿跂床悬脚，久成血痹，足重腰疼。凡脚汗勿入水，作骨痹，亦作遁痓。久忍小便，脉冷，兼成冷痹。

Don't take off clothes immediately after sweating; otherwise, people are likely to suffer from hemiplegia. Don't expose head to the wind right after taking a bath; otherwise, they are likely to suffer from leprosy and thorn wind disease. Don't face fire immediately after exposing in cold weather; otherwise, they are likely to suffer from epilepsy, dizziness and headache. Don't sit by the bed with feet hanging; otherwise, they are likely to suffer from blood−arthralgia over time, resulting in heavy foot and lumbago. Don't dip feet in cold water with feet sweating; otherwise, they are likely to suffer from bone disease and latent chronic diseases. Don't hold urine for a long time; otherwise, they are likely to suffer from cold vessel and cold arthralgia.

凡食热物汗出勿荡风，发疰头痛，令人目涩饶睡。凡欲眠勿歌咏，不祥。眠起勿大语，损人气。

Those who sweat after eating hot food should avoid facing wind; otherwise, they are likely to suffer from headache, dry eye and somnolence. Those who are ready for sleep should avoid singing, for it is ominous. Those who just wake up should avoid speaking aloud, for it hurts Yang Qi.

凡飞鸟投人不可食，鸟若开口及毛下有疮，并不可食之。凡热泔洗头，冷水濯，成头风。凡人卧，头边勿安火炉，令人头重、目赤、鼻干。凡卧讫，头旁勿安灯，令人六神不安。冬日温足冻脑，

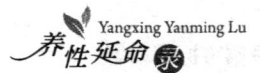

春秋脑足俱冻，此乃圣人之常法也。

Don't eat any bird that flies into your arms, or those with sores under the feather. Don't rinse hair with cold water after washing with hot rice soup, which leads to head wind disease. Don't put a stove beside head when sleep, which leads to heavy head, red eye and dry nose. Don't switch the light on when sleep, which makes one uneasy. It is the sage's way of health preservation to warm foot while cool head in winter, and cool both head and foot in spring and autumn.

凡新哭泣讫便食，即成气病。夜卧勿覆头，妇人勿跂灶坐，大忌。凡唾不用远，远即成肺病，令人手重、背疼、咳嗽。凡人魇，勿点灯照，定魇死，暗唤之即吉，亦不可近前及急唤。

Don't eat immediately after crying, which leads to Qi-related disease. Don't bury head in quilt when sleeping at night. It is a big taboo to sit on the stove for women. Don't spit too far away, which leads to lung disease, and causes heavy hands, back pain and cough. If anyone has a nightmare in sleep, don't light the lamp; otherwise he will be indelibly killed . Just call him quietly and avoid shouting nearby or urgently.

凡人卧勿开口，久成病渴，并失血色。凡且起勿以冷水开目洗面，令人目涩、失明、饶泪。凡行途中触热，逢河勿洗面，生乌奸。人睡讫忽觉，勿饮水更卧，成水痹。

Don't sleep with mouth open, which leads to thirst and pale face. Don't wash face with cold water when get up in the morning, which leads to dry eye, blindness and hyperdacryosis. Don't wash face in river water when heated in journey, which leads to taches noir. Don't lie down again after drinking water when suddenly wake up from sleep, which leads to water arthralgia.

凡时病新汗解，勿饮冷水，损人心腹，不平复。凡空腹不可见闻臭尸气，入鼻令人成病。凡欲见死尸，皆须先饮酒及咬蒜，辟毒气。凡小儿不用令指月，两耳后生疮欲断，名月蚀疮，捣蝦蟆末傅即差，并别余疮并不生。凡产妇不可见狐臭人，能令产妇著肿。

Don't drink cold water just recovering from seasonal diseases, which damages heart and abdomen, leading to obstinateness of disease. Don't look or smell the odor of corpse on an empty stomach, which makes people sick in case of smelling. Anyone who is going to see a dead body must first drink alcohol and chew garlic to avoid poisonous gas. Children should not point to the moon with fingers, which might lead to opisthotic sores, known as lunar eclipse sore. It can be treated

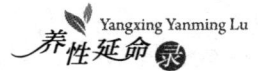

by smearing some toad powder, which may prevent from causing other sores. Pregnant women should not meet those with hircismus, which leads to edema.

凡人卧不用于窗櫺下，令人六神不安。凡卧，春夏欲得头向东，秋冬头向西，有所利益。凡丈夫，饥欲得坐小便，饱则立小便，令人无病。凡人睡，欲得屈膝侧卧，益人气力。凡卧，欲得数转侧，语笑欲令至少，莫令声高大。

Don't sleep under the window, which makes people uneasy. When sleeping, it is healthy to point head to the East in spring and summer, and to the West in autumn and winter. When a man is hungry, he should squat to urinate, and when he is full, he should stand to urinate, which can prevent people from getting sick. When sleep, people should bend knees and lie on sides, which can increase their strength. When lying down, they should frequently turn over, talk and laugh as little as possible, and not speak aloud.

春欲得暝卧早起，夏秋欲得夜卧早起，冬欲得早卧晏起，皆有所益。虽云早起，莫在鸡鸣前，晏起莫在日出后。冬日天地闭，阳气藏，人不欲作劳出汗，发泄阳气，损人。

In spring, people should go to sleep after dark and get up early;

in summer and autumn, people should go to bed late and get up early; in winter, people should go to bed early and get up late. It is good for health. Don't get up before cockcrow or after sunrise. In winter, when heaven and earth are not as active and Yang Qi stores inside, people should not work to sweat, which discharges Yang Qi and damages the body.

新沐浴讫，勿当风结髻，勿以湿头卧，使人患头风，眩闷、发秃、面肿、齿痛、耳聋。湿衣及汗衣皆不可著久，令发疮及患风瘙痒。

Don't wear hair in a bun in the wind right after washing head or taking a bath, and don't sleep with hair wet, which leads to head wind, dizziness, chest tightness, baldness, swollen face, toothache and deafness. Don't wear wet or sweaty clothes for a long time, which leads to sore, rheumatism and pruritus.

老君曰：正月旦，中庭向寅地再拜，咒曰："（某甲）年年受大道之恩，太清玄门，愿还（某甲）去岁之年。男女皆三通自咒。常行此道，延年（玄女有清神之法，淮南有祠灶之规，咸欲体合真灵，护生者也）。

Lao Tsu tells us to bow respectfully to the Northeast twice in the

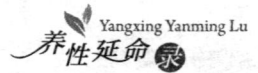

atrium on the first day of the first month （lunar calendar）, and says: He （using one's name） receives the grace of the Dao every year and rejuvenates himself. Both men and women repeat the incantation three times by themselves oftentimes, which helps to prolong their life. （The goddess of the Ninth Heaven has the method of purifying her mind, and Liu An, the king of Huainan, has the rules of sacrificing the kitchen god. Both of them require the unity of body and true spirit to protect life.）

《仙经秘要》：常存念心中，有气大如鸡子，内赤外黄，辟众邪延年也。欲却众邪百鬼，常存念为炎火如斗，煌煌光明，则百邪不敢干人，可入瘟疫之中。暮卧常存作赤气在外，白气在内，以覆身，辟众邪鬼魅。

*Xianjing Miyao*（*The Secret of Immortal Classic*）says: If people often think that there is an air mass as big as an egg in heart, red inside and yellow outside, it can help to avoid all kinds of evils and prolong life. If people often think that there is a ball of fire in heart, it can help to avoid all kinds of demons and ghosts, and various evils cannot invade the body, even in a plague. When sleeping at night, if people often think that there is red Qi outside and white Qi inside to cover the whole body, it can help to avoid all kinds of demons and ghosts.

老君曰：凡人求道，勿犯五逆六不祥，有犯者凶。大小便向西一逆，向北二逆，向日三逆，向月四逆，仰视天及星辰五逆。夜起裸形一不祥，旦起嗔恚二不祥，向灶骂詈三不祥，以足向火四不祥，夫妻昼合五不祥，怨恚师父六不祥。

Lao Tzu says: Those who seek Dao should avoid the five taboos and six kinds of ominousness, or it will be dangerous. When defecating, it is unwise to face the west, the north, the sun, the moon, and the heaven. It is ominous to get up naked at night, be angry in the morning, curse at the stove, stretch feet to fire, have sex at daytime, and resent masters.

凡人旦起恒言善事，天与之福，勿言奈何，歌啸，名曰请祸。慎勿上床卧歌，凶。始卧伏床，凶。饮食伏床，凶。以匙箸击盘上，凶。司阴之神，在人口左，人有阴祸，司阴白之于天，天则考人魂魄。司杀之神，在人口右，人有恶言，司杀白之于司命，司命记之，罪满即杀。二神监口，惟向人求非，安可不慎言？舌者，身之兵革，善恶由之而生，故道家所忌。

Heaven blesses everyone who gets up in the morning and always says good things; those who say helpless things or sing loudly will cause troubles, known as "invite misfortune". It is

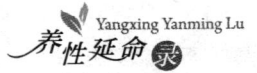

ominous to sing while lying on bed, or be in prone position right after lying on bed, or eat and drink on bed. It is also ominous to knock on the plate with spoon and chopsticks. The god in charge of hell, on the left of people's mouth, will tell divinity if people hurt others and they will be interrogated with torture; the god in charge of killing, on the right of people's mouth, will tell the god in charge of life if people say vicious words, and he in turn records and kills them when records are sufficient enough. There are two gods guarding both sides of mouth, finding fault with people who make mistakes, so how can you speak carelessly! The tongue is a weapon that causes people to kill themselves. The good and evil are produced by the tongue, so practitioners are cautious with it.

饮玉泉者，令人延年，除百病。玉泉者，口中唾也。鸡鸣、平旦、日中、日晡、黄昏、夜半时，一日一夕，凡七漱玉泉食之，每食辄满口咽之，延年。

Those who swallow jade spring can prolong life and eliminate all diseases. Jade spring is the saliva in people's mouth. If people swallow saliva with mouth full seven times a day at cockcrow, daybreak, noon, late afternoon, dusk, and midnight, they can prolong their life.

发，血之穷；齿，骨之穷；爪，筋之穷。千过梳发，发不白；朝夕啄齿，齿不龋；爪不数截，筋不替。人常数欲照镜，谓之存形，形与神相存，此其意也。若矜容颜色自爱玩，不如勿照。

Hair is the tip of blood, teeth are the tip of bone, and nails are the tip of tendons. If people comb their hair a thousand times, their hair will not whitening; if people tap teeth oftentimes, their teeth will not decayed; if people don't cut fingernails, their tendons will not grow. People should often look in the mirror, known as "keep in shape", so that the body and spirit can support each other. But if people pity or admire themselves in the mirror, it's certainly not admirable.

凡人常以正月一日、二月二日、三月三日、四月八日、五月一日、六月二十七日、七月十一日、八月八日、九月二十一日、十月十四日、十一月十一日、十二月三十日，但常以此日取枸杞菜，煮作汤沐浴，令人光泽，不病不老。月蚀宜救，活人除殃。活万人，与天同功（天不好杀，圣人则之。不好杀者，是助天地长养，故招胜福）。善梦可说，恶梦默之，则养性延年也。

People who take a bath with wolfberry boiled water on January 1, February 2, March 3, April 8, May 1, June 27, July 11, August 8, September 21, October 14, November 11 and December 30, can make their skin shiny and avoid illness and aging. In the event of a lunar

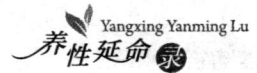

eclipse, people can save lives and eliminate disasters, and they are as great as the heaven if they save thousands（Heaven does not like killing, and saints follow the rule, which help heaven and earth to grow all things, so it can lead to great blessings）. Good dreams can be spoken out while horrible ones should be held back, which can prolong life.

# 服气疗病篇第四

## Chapter 4　Moving Qi for Treatment

《元阳经》曰：常以鼻纳气，含而漱满，舌料唇齿咽之，一日一夜得千咽甚佳。当少饮食，饮食多则气逆，百脉闭。百脉闭则气不行，气不行则生病。

*Yuanyang Jing*（*Yuanyang Classic*）says: It is good to inhale fresh air through the nose, hold it to rinse mouth until there is enough saliva, and stir the lips to swallow it. It is healthy to repeat this process for a thousand times a day and night. People should eat less because too much can cause Qi counterflow and thus meridians of the whole body are blocked. The blockage of meridians will cause Qi movement disorder, which in turn causes diseases.

《玄示》曰：志者，气之帅也；气者，体之充也。善者遂其

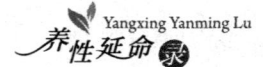

生，恶者丧其形。故行气之法，少食自节，动其形，和其气血。因轻而止之，勿过失突，复而还之，其状若咽。正体端形，心意专一，固守中外，上下俱闭，神周形骸，调畅四溢，修守关元，满而足实，因之而众邪自出。

*Xuanshi*（*Explanation of the Emperor Huang and Lao Tzu's Canon*）says: Will is the commander that guides the movement of Qi in the body, and Qi constitutes the body and makes it strong. Those who are good at moving Qi can prolong their life, while those who aren't will injure the body. Therefore, the proper way to move Qi is to reduce diet, exercise the body and calm Qi and blood. People should move Qi in a mild way to avoid excess or deficiency. This process should be repeated many times, just like swallowing saliva. Sit upright and concentrate the mind, secure Qi inside and outside the body and block all the upper and lower openings. In this way, Qi runs over the whole body and moves smoothly and freely. If people exercise Guanyuan point（CV4）, they will be energetic and healthy, and all pathogenic Qi will go out of the body.

彭祖曰：常闭气纳息，从平旦至日中，乃跪坐拭目，摩搦身体，舐唇咽唾，服气数十，乃起行言笑。其偶有疲倦不安，便导引闭气，以攻所患，必存其身头面、九窍、五脏、四肢，至于发端，皆令所在觉其气云行体中，起于鼻口，下达十指末，则澄和真神，不须针药灸刺。凡行气，欲除百病，随所在作念之。头痛念头，足痛念足，和气往攻之，从时至时，便自消矣。时气中冷，可闭气以取汗，汗出辄周身则解矣。

Peng Zu says: It is good to hold breath and breathe out from dawn to noon frequently. Only then can you kneel and wipe your eyes, massage your body, lick your lips, swallow saliva, and take your breath dozens of times before standing up to walk or talk with others. If you feel tired and out of sorts occasionally, you can guide your breath with will and hold your breath to make Qi reach the affected area, and let Qi run all over your body, from head, face, nine orifices to the five zang-organs and four limbs, and then to the end of hair. You will feel Qi like cloud floating in your body, starting from your nose and mouth, and reaching the end of your fingers. In this way, the spirit will be refreshed as clear as water, and there will be no disease. There is no need for medical treatment such as medicine, acupuncture and moxibustion. If you want to treat all kinds of diseases through Qi moving, you should visualize with your mind to move Qi to the place where the pain is located. If the pain is located in head, concentrate your mind on head; if the pain is located in foot, concentrate your mind on foot. Thus, Qi is conducted by mind to treat the disease. With the passage of time, the

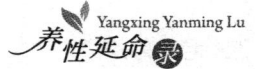

pain will be eliminated gradually. If you are attacked by pathogenic cold due to seasonal changes, method of blocking Qi can be used for sweating, and you will recover from sweating.

行气闭气，虽是治身之要，然当先达解其理趣。又宜空虚，不可饱满。若气有结滞，不得空流，或致疮疖，譬如泉源不可壅遏。若食生鱼、生菜、肥肉，及喜怒忧恚不除，而以行气，令人发上气。凡欲学行气，皆当以渐。

Although moving and blocking Qi are the key points of health preservation, we should first understand its mechanism. The intestines and stomach should be empty, not full. If Qi and blood are stagnant and do not flow smoothly, people may suffer from sores and boils, just like a spring, which cannot be blocked. If you move Qi when eating raw fish, lettuce, fat meat or when you are not calm in emotions, Qi will counterflow. Anyone who wants to learn the method of moving Qi should do it step by step.

刘君安曰：食生吐死，可以长存，谓鼻纳气为生，口吐气为死也。凡人不能服气，从朝至暮常习不息，徐而舒之，但令鼻纳口吐，所谓吐故纳新也。

Liu An says: Inhale fresh air and exhale stale air, so that people can prolong their life. This means that the fresh air inhaled by the nose is the Qi for health while the stale air exhaled by the mouth is the Qi for disease. If people can't move Qi, practice from morning to night to make their breathing slow and comfortable. As long as people inhale fresh air through their nose and exhale stale air through mouth, their life can be preserved. This is called "exhaling the stale and inhaling the fresh".

《服气经》曰：道者，气也。保气则得道，得道则长存。神者，精也。保精则神明，神明则长生。精者，血脉之川流，守骨之灵神也。精去则骨枯，骨枯则死矣。是以为道，务宝其精。

*Fuqi Jing* ( *Classic of Moving Qi* ) says: Dao is genuine Qi. If people can preserve genuine Qi, they can get Dao, and they in turn can live long. Spirit is the essence. If people can maintain the essence, they can have spiritual clarity, which in turn can make one live for a long time. The essence is like the stream of blood, the divinity guarding the bones. Loss of essence will lead to withering bones, and then to death. Therefore, if people pursue Dao, they must cherish essence like treasures.

从夜半到日中为生气，从日中后至夜半为死气，当以生气时

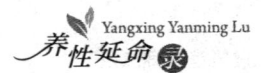
正偃卧，瞑目握固（握固者，如婴儿之拳手，以四指押拇指也），闭气不息，于心中数至二百，乃口吐气出之。日增息，如此身神具，五脏安，能闭气至二百五十，华盖明。华盖明则耳目聪明，举身无病，邪不干人也。

The period from midnight to noon is dominated by Yang Qi, and the period from noon to midnight is dominated by Yin Qi. When Yang is growing, people should lie on the back, close the eyes, clench the fist like a baby holding thumb with four fingers, hold breath and count to 200 in the heart before spitting out Qi from the mouth. Increase the period of meditation every day; in doing so, the body and mind will be healthy and the five zang−organs will be peaceful. If people can hold breath to 250, the eyebrows will shine, they can hear and see better, and thus they are healthy and pathogenic Qi cannot invade them.

凡行气，以鼻纳气，以口吐气，微而引之，名曰长息。纳气有一，吐气有六。纳气一者，谓吸也；吐气六者，谓吹、呼、唏、呵、嘘、呬，皆出气也。

When moving Qi, people should take in with the nose and breathe out with the mouth, so that the breath becomes slight and gradually longer, which is known as "long breath". There is one way to inhale while six ways to exhale. Inhaling is the only way to take in Qi while blowing, expiring, sighing, puffing, hissing and panting are ways to breathe Qi out.

凡人之息，一呼一吸，元有此数。欲为长息吐气之法，时寒可吹，温可呼，委曲治病，吹以去热，呼以去风，唏以去烦，呵以下气，嘘以散滞，呬以解极。

All people breathe in and out rhythmically, which is the basic law of respiration. However, long breath can be employed for treatment. Generally speaking, blowing method can be used when the weather is cold and the expiring method is used when the weather is warm. Different methods should be used for various conditions: Blowing can remove the diseases caused by pathogenic heat, expiring can remove the diseases caused by pathogenic wind, signing can remove the boredom and annoyance in the heart, puffing can make the Qi descend, hissing can dissolve the stagnant Qi, and panting can relieve extreme fatigue.

凡人极者，则多嘘呬。道家行气，率不欲嘘呬。嘘呬者长息之心也。此男女俱存法，法出于《仙经》。行气者，先除鼻中毛，所谓通神之路。若天恶风猛、大寒大热时，勿取气。

When people are extremely tired, they often hiss and pant.

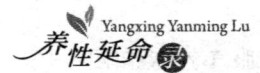

However, most Taoists do not use these two methods. These two methods are important for long breath and can be maintained by both men and women. Those methods come from *Xianjing* ( *Immortal Classic* ). Those who practice Qi must first remove the hair in their nose, which is called opening the way to communicate with divinity. But remember: Do not move Qi in bad weather, strong wind, or extreme conditions.

《明医论》云：疾之所起，自生五劳，五劳既用，二脏先损，心肾受邪，腑脏俱病。五劳者：一曰志劳，二曰思劳，三曰心劳，四曰忧劳，五曰疲劳。五劳则生六极：一曰气极，二曰血极，三曰筋极，四曰骨极，五曰精极，六曰髓极。六极即为七伤，七伤故变为七痛，七痛为病，令人邪气多正气少，忽忽喜怒悲伤，不乐饮食，不生肌肤，颜色无泽，发白枯槁，甚者令人得大风偏枯筋缩，四肢拘急挛缩，百关隔塞，羸瘦短气，腰脚疼痛。此由早娶，用精过差，血气不足，极劳之所致也。

*Mingyi Lun* ( *Famous Doctor's Discussion* ) says: The occurrence of diseases is caused by five kinds of strain. When the five kinds of strain injure the body, they first damage the heart and kidney, which in turn affect the other viscera. The five kinds of strain are: will overstrain, pensiveness overstrain, heart overstrain, anxiety overstrain, and fatigue, which lead to six kinds of extreme weakness of Qi, blood, muscle, bone, essence and marrow. The six kinds of extreme weakness in turn cause seven injuries or impairments. When seven impairments cause diseases, pathogenic Qi is exuberant while healthy Qi is deficient and thus symptoms occur like unstable mood, loss of appetite, coarse skin, dull complexion, white and withering hair, and even hemiplegia, spasm of limbs, obstruction of body orifices, emaciation, shortness of breath, waist and foot pain. All of this are caused by overconsumption of semen due to early marriage, insufficient Qi and blood, and extreme fatigue.

凡病之来，不离于五脏，事须识相。若不识者，勿为之耳。心脏病者，体有冷热，呼吹二气出之；肺脏病者，胸膈胀满，嘘气出之；脾脏病者，体上游风习习，身痒疼闷，唏气出之。肝脏病者，眼疼，愁忧不乐，呵气出之。

The causes of diseases are always related to the five zang-organs. Diagnosis is always necessary before treatment, and if you don't know the disease, don't treat it blindly. If there is a heart disease, there are cold and heat pathogens in the body, which can be discharged by "expiring" and "blowing". If there is a lung disease, there is distension and fullness in the chest and abdomen, which can be discharged by "hissing". If there is a spleen disease, there is

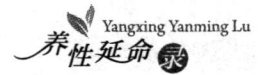
wandering pain, itching, and stuffy pain around the whole body, which can be discharged by "signing". If there is a liver disease, there is pain in the eyes and anxiety in emotion, which can be discharged by "puffing".

已上十二种调气法，但常以鼻引气，口中吐气，当令气声逐字吹呼嘘呵唏呬吐之。若患者依此法，皆须恭敬用心为之，无有不差，此即愈病长生要术也。

For the above twelve methods of regulating Qi, people should often inhale through the nose and exhale through the mouth. When exhaling, people should follow the order of blowing, expiring, hissing, puffing, signing and panting. If patients are treated in this way, they should first do these respectfully and carefully. If so, there is no disease that cannot be cured. This is the way to cure the disease and prolong life.

# 导引按摩篇第五

## Chapter 5　Conduction Exercise and Tuina

《导引经》云：清旦未起，啄齿二七，闭目握固，漱满唾，三咽。气寻闭而不息自极，极乃徐徐出气，满三止。

*Daoyin Jing*（*Conduction Classic*）says: Before you get up in the morning, tap teeth 14 times, close eyes and hold hands firmly. Rinse saliva in the mouth and swallow it three times when the saliva is full. Hold your breath and exhale slowly until you can't manage it, and repeat this process three times.

便起，狼踞鸱顾，左右自摇曳，不息自极，复三。便起下床，握固不息，顿踵三还，上一手，下一手，亦不息自极三。又叉手项上，左右自了捩，不息复三。又伸两足及叉手前却自极，复三。

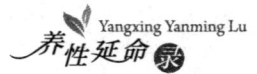
皆当朝暮为之，能数尤善。平旦以两掌相摩令热，熨眼三过。次又以指按目四眦，令人目明。

Then get up, squat like a wolf, and twist left and right like an owl. Hold your breath and exhale until you can't manage it, and repeat this process three times. Then get up and go to the ground, hold your hands firmly, hold your breath, stand on tiptoe and tap the ground three times. Raise one hand and press the other, and interchange between the right and left, hold your breath and exhale until you can't manage it, and repeat this process three times. Then cross your hands, hold your neck back, twist left and right, hold your breath and do it three times. Then stretch out your feet, cross your hands, stretch forward as far as possible and withdraw, and repeat three times. You should practice the whole process in the morning and evening and it's better to repeat it more times. Rub your hands together at dawn and cover your eyes with your hands three times, and then rub your fingers around your eyes, which can make your eyes bright.

按经文，拘魂门，制魄户，名曰握固，与魂魄安门户也。此固精明目，留年还魄之法，若能终日握之，邪气百毒不得入。

It also says that holding fingers firmly with your thumb inside is beneficial for soul, which is like installing a gate for the entry and exit of the soul. This is the way to strengthen the essence, brighten the eyes, prolong the life, and calm the soul. If you do this all day, pathogenic Qi can't invade your body.

《内解》云：一曰精，二曰唾，三曰泪，四曰涕，五曰汗，六曰溺，皆所以损人也，但为损者有轻重耳。人能终日不涕唾，随有漱满咽之，若恒含枣核咽之，令人爱气生津液，此大要也（谓取津液，非咽核也）。常每旦啄齿三十六通，能至三百弥佳，令人齿坚不痛。次则以舌搅漱口中津液，满口咽之，三过止。

*Neijie* ( *Yin's Explanation of Lao Tsu* ) says: Disorder of semen, saliva, tears, nasal discharge, sweat and urine can impair the body, whether light or heavy. If people don't shed tears or spit the whole day, but instead rinse the saliva in mouth at any time, and then swallow it when it is full, just as they have jujube pit in the mouth to stimulate saliva secretion and swallow it, it can help people maintain original Qi and generate fluid. This is an important way of health preservation ( Here what we mean is rinsing the saliva rather than eating jujube pit ). If people tap teeth 36 times every morning — it will be better to tap 300 times — the teeth will be strengthened and toothache will be avoided. Then stir the saliva in mouth with tongue to make it full, then swallow it, and repeat it three times.

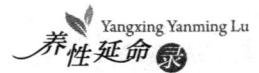

次摩指少阳令热，以熨目，满二七止，令人目明。每旦初起，以两手掩两耳，极上下热揉之，二七止，令人耳不聋。次又啄齿漱玉泉三咽，缩鼻闭气，右手从头上引左耳二七，复以左手从头上引右耳二七止，令人延年不聋。次又引两鬓发举之一七，则总取发两手向上，极势抬上一七，令人血气通，头不白。

Rub the side of the ring finger close to the little finger to make your hand warm and cover your eyes with hands, and repeat it 14 times, which can make your eyes bright. When you get up every morning, cover your ears with your hands, rub up and down 14 times to make them warm, which makes you avoid deaf. Then tap your teeth, rinse the saliva in your mouth and swallow it three times successively, hold your nose and don't breathe, pull the left ear 14 times with your right hand around your head, and then pull the right ear 14 times with your left hand around your head, which can prolong your life and keep your ears from deafness. Pull the hair on both temples up 7 times, then hold all the hair with both hands and pull it up 7 times, which can smooth both Qi and blood, and avoid hair whitening.

又法：摩手令热，以摩面，从上至下，去邪气，令人面上有光彩。又法：摩手令热，摩身体，从上至下，名曰干浴，令人胜风寒时气热，头痛百病皆除。夜欲卧时，常以两手揩摩身体，名曰干浴，辟风邪。峻坐，以左手托头，仰右手向上尽势托，以身并手振动三，右手托头振动亦三，除人睡闷。

Another way: rub your hands warm and massage your face from up to down to remove pathogenic Qi and make your face shiny. A third way: rub your hands and massage your body from up to down, known as "dry bath", which can dispel the wind-cold and pathogenic heat, meanwhile, headache and other diseases can also be cured. Before going to bed at night, rub your body with hands, known as "dry bath", which can ward off pathogenic wind. Sit upright, hold your head with your left hand, lift the palm of your right hand upward, and vibrate your body and hands three times; then change the right hand to hold the head, repeat the above action and vibrate three times to eliminate chest stuffiness in sleep.

平旦日未出前，面向南峻坐，两手托胜，尽势振动三，令人面有光泽生。且起未梳洗前，峻坐，以左手握右手于左胜上，前却尽热接左胜三；又以右手握左手于右胜上，前却接右胜亦三；次又两手向前，尽势推三；次又叉两手向胸前，以两肘向前，尽势三；次直引左臂，卷曲右臂，如挽一斛五斗弓势，尽力为之，右手挽弓势，亦然。

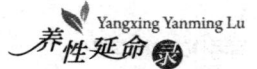

Before sunrise in the morning, sit upright facing south, hold your thighs with both hands and try to vibrate three times to make your face glorious and shiny. Before grooming in the morning, sit upright, hold right hand with left hand and put them on left thigh, lean forward and rub left leg three times; then hold left hand with right hand and put them on right leg, lean forward and rub right leg three times; push palms forward three times with both hands, cross hands in front of chest and extend elbows forward three times; lift left arm straight and the right arm bent, and try to pull it apart like pulling a heavy bow, and repeat the action the other way round.

次以右手托地，左手仰托天，尽势，右亦然；次卷两手，向前筑各三七；次卷左手尽势向背上，握指三，右手亦如之；疗背膊臂肘劳气。数为之弥佳。

Then press the ground with right hand and lift left hand up as far as possible, and repeat the same action with the right hand. Hold two fists and strike forward 21 times like knocking on a building. Hold left hand toward back and clench fingers three times, and repeat this action with right hand. This method can treat back, arm and elbow injuries, and the more the better.

平旦便转讫，以一长拄杖策腋，垂左脚于床前，徐峻，尽势擎左脚五七回，右亦如之。疗脚气、疼闷，腰肾冷气、冷痹及膝冷，并主之。日夕三擎弥佳。勿大饱及忍小便，擎如不用拄杖，但遣所擎脚不着地，手扶一物亦得。晨夕梳头满一千梳，大去头风，令人发不白。梳讫，以盐花及生麻油搓头顶上弥佳。如有神明膏搓之，甚佳。

After the dawn activity, lean on armpit with a long stick, hang left foot in front of bed, and slowly try to lift left foot 35 times, and then repeat this with the right foot. It can treat beriberi, pain, dysphoria, cold waist and kidney, cold arthralgia and cold knee. It's better to pull it three times a day, but remember don't push it when you're full or have urine. If you don't want a stick, you can hold something with your hand as long as the foot doesn't fall to the ground. Comb your hair a thousand times in the morning and evening, and this can remove head wind and avoid hair whitening. After combing your hair, it's better to rub your head with a pinch of salt and raw sesame oil, and Shenming Gao（Ointment for mind）is best.

且欲梳洗时，叩齿一百六十，随有津液便咽之。讫，以水漱口，又更以盐末揩齿，即含取微酢清浆半小合许，熟漱。取盐汤吐洗两目讫，以冷水洗面，不得遣冷水入眼中。此法齿得坚净，目明

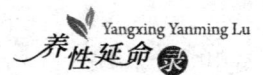
无泪，永无蠿齿。平旦洗面时漱口讫，咽一两咽冷水，令人心明净，去胸臆中热。

Before grooming in the morning, tap teeth 160 times and swallow saliva in mouth. After that, rinse mouth with water, wipe teeth with salt, and then gargle repeatedly with light vinegar. Then spit out the salt water to wash eyes, wash face with cold water and avoid cold water entering the eyes. This method can make teeth firm and clean, eyes clear without turbidity, and you will never suffer from dental caries. When washing face at dawn, rinse mouth and swallow one or two mouthfuls of cold water to clear your heart and remove the pathogenic heat.

谯国华佗善养性，弟子广陵吴普、彭城樊阿授术于佗。佗尝语普曰：人体欲得劳动，但不当使极耳。人身常摇动，则谷气消，血脉流通，病不生。譬犹户枢不朽是也。古之仙者及汉时有道士君倩者，为导引之术，作熊经鸱顾，引挽腰体，动诸关节，以求难老也。

Hua Tuo is good at health preservation. His disciples Wu Pu and Fan E learned health preservation from him. Hua Tuo once told Wu Pu that people needs activity, but they can't overwork. With regular physical activity, the nutrition of grains can be digested and absorbed, blood can circulate smoothly, and thus no disease occurs. It is just like a rolling stone gathers no moss. Ancient immortals and a Taoist named Jun Qian in the Han Dynasty created the art of conduction exercise, imitating the movements of bear climbing branches and owl looking around to stretch their waist and move their joints, so as to delay aging.

吾有一术，名曰五禽戏：一曰虎，二曰鹿，三曰熊，四曰猿，五曰鸟，亦以除疾，兼利手足，以常导引。体中不快，因起作一禽之戏，遣微汗出即止，以粉涂身，即身体轻便，腹中思食。吴普行之，年九十余岁，耳目聪明，牙齿坚完，吃食如少壮也。

I have a set of health preservation techniques called five-animal exercise. These five animals are tiger, deer, bear, monkey and bird. It can be used not only to cure diseases, but also to facilitate hands and feet. I often use this technique to conduct my body. If you feel unwell, get up and do one of those exercises, stop when the body sweats slightly. If you smear the body with powder, you will feel light and have the appetite to eat. Wu Pu exercised like this. In his nineties, he could still hear and see clearly, his teeth were strong and complete, and he ate like a young man.

虎戏者，四肢距地，前三掷，却二掷，长引腰，侧脚仰天，

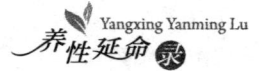

即返距行，前、却各七过也。鹿戏者，四肢距地，引项反顾，左三右二，左右伸脚，伸缩亦三亦二也。熊戏者，正仰以两手抱膝下，举头，左擗地七，右亦七，蹲地，以手左右托地。猿戏者，攀物自悬，伸缩身体，上下一七，以脚拘物自悬，左右七，手钩却立，按头各七。鸟戏者，双立手，翘一足，伸两臂，扬眉用力，各二七，坐伸脚，手挽足距各七，缩伸二臂各七也。夫五禽戏法，任力为之，以汗出为度，有汗以粉涂身，消谷食，益气力，除百病，能存行之者，必得延年。

The tiger-exercise is to touch the ground with both hands and feet, jump forward three times, and then backward twice, stretch the waist and feet and face the sky, crawl with four limbs to move forward and backward seven times respectively. The deer-exercise is to touch the ground with both hands and feet, stretch the neck and look back, three times on the left and twice on the right; stretch the left foot three times and the right foot twice. The bear-exercise is to lie on the back, hold knees with both hands, raise head to the left and hammer the ground with head seven times, and also seven times to the right; squat on the ground and press the ground with both hands. The monkey-exercise is to climb an object to suspend the body, and stretch the body up and down seven times. Hook the object upside down with both feet, and exchange feet to suspend the body seven times respectively. Then hook the object with hands and retreat to stand, and press head seven times with left and right hands respectively. The bird-exercise is to erect both palms, raise one foot, stretch both arms, raise the eyebrows, and do with force 14 times for the left and right foot respectively. Then sit down to stretch the feet forward, pull the left and right toes seven times, and stretch arms seven times. To practice the five-animal exercise, people need to act according to their physical conditions. They should stop when sweat appears and smear the body with powder after that. This five-animal exercise can help digestion, increase strength and eliminate various diseases. Those who can keep exercising are bound to prolong their life.

又有法：安坐，未食前自按摩，以两手相叉，伸臂股，导引诸脉，胜于汤药。正坐，仰天呼出，饮食醉饱之气立消。夏天为之，令人凉矣。

There is another way of health preservation. Sit down quietly and do self-massage before eating. Cross hands and fingers and stretch forward together with legs, which can dredge all meridians. The effect is better than that of herbal medicine. Sit upright and exhale, and the turbid Qi caused by eating and drinking will dissipate immediately. If you do this in summer, it will make you cool.

# 御女损益篇第六

## Chapter 6　Benefits and Harms of Sex

道以精为宝，施之则生人，留之则生身。生身则求度在仙位，生人则功遂而身退。功遂而身退，则陷欲以为剧，何况妄施而废弃，损不觉多，故疲劳而命堕。天地有阴阳，阴阳人所贵，贵之合于道，但当慎无费。

Dao regards the essence as treasure. The discharge of semen can give birth to children while the preservation of that can help to maintain the body. The maintenance of the body can help to pursue immortality, while libido should be restrained after giving birth to children. It is wrong to immerse in desire excessively. Immoderate sex and discharge of semen can unknowingly increase the damage to human body and even lead to fatigue and death. There is Yin and Yang for earth and heaven, and they interact with each other. Thus, it is natural and important for humans to have sex. What is significant is following the rule and avoiding the waste of essence.

彭祖曰：上士别床，中士异被。服药千裹，不如独卧。色使目盲，声使耳聋，味使口爽。苟能节宣其道，适抑扬其通塞者，可以增寿。

Peng Zu says: People who live a long life often sleep in a different bed with their wife, while those who know health preservation do not share the same quilt with their wife. Taking a thousand doses of medicine for longevity is no better than sleeping alone. Diverse colors dazzle people, various music makes people deaf, and delicious food weakens people's taste. If we understand the truth of abstinence and discharge and achieve the harmony between them, we can prolong our life.

一日之忌，暮食无饱（夜饱食眠，损一日之寿）；一月之忌，暮饮无醉（夜醉卧，损一月之寿）；一岁之忌，暮须远内（一交损一岁之寿，养之不复）；终身之忌，暮须护气（暮卧习闭口，开口失气，又邪从口入）。

One day's taboo is to be excessively full with dinner（sleeping with full stomach at night will make one lose one day's life）, one

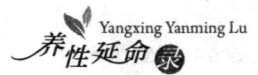

month's taboo is to be drunk at night （sleeping with drunkenness at night will make one lose one month's life）, one year's taboo is to be immersed in sex at night （one-time intercourse will make one lose one year's life, which cannot be recuperated with nourishment）, and a lifelong taboo is to waste Qi at night （it is beneficial to develop the habit of closing mouth when sleeping at night, or Qi will be lost and body will be invaded with mouth open）.

采女问彭祖曰：人年六十，当闭精守一，为可尔否？

A fairy named Cai Nü asks Peng Zu: When people are 60 years old, should they always curb their semen from discharging? Is it true?

彭祖曰：不然。男不欲无女，无女则意动，意动则神劳，神劳则损寿。若念真正无可思而大佳，然而万一焉。有强郁闭之，难持易失，使人漏精尿浊，以致鬼交之病。

Peng Zu says: This is not the case. Men can't live without women, or they often think about sexual desire. Strong sexual desire leads to mental fatigue, which in turn reduce their life expectancy. It is best for people to be pure without any desire; however, there is almost no one in 10000 people. Some people force themselves to keep semen from discharging, but in fact, it is difficult to hold it full but easy to discharge, which makes semen leak and urine turbid, and finally have obscene dreams at night.

又欲令气未感动，阳道垂弱，欲以御女者，先摇动令其强起，但徐徐接之，令得阴气，阴气推之，须臾自强，强而用之，务令迟疏。精动而正闭精，缓息瞑目，偃卧导引，身体更复，可御他女。欲一动则辄易人，易人可长生。

When Yang Qi that inspires libido does not exert force, the penis is in a flaccid state. If he wants sexual intercourse, he should first shake the penis to make it strong and erectile, and slowly insert it into the vagina to make it respond the Yin Qi of a woman. With the function of woman's Yin Qi, it will naturally be strong before long. When it is becoming strong, he should use it in a slow and gentle way. When semen is induced, he should take a right attitude toward sex, lock the semen, slow the breath down, slightly close eyes and lie on the back to conduct the body. Only after the body recovers can he have sex with other women. As soon as libido starts, he can repeat the process, which can prolong his life.

若御一女，阴气既微，为益亦少。又阳道法火，阴道法水。水能制火，阴亦消阳，久用不止，阴气吸阳，阳则转损，所得

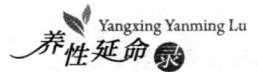

不补所失。但能御十二女子而复不泄者，令人老有美色。若御九十三女而不泄者，年万岁。

If a man has sex with only one woman, he can benefit little from it because her Yin Qi has declined. In addition, man is like fire and woman is like water. Water can restrain fire, the same is true of Yin and Yang. Having sex with a woman for a long time, the man will be impaired because Yin Qi consumes Yang Qi and thus Yang declines, and the benefits the man obtained can't equal the losses caused. If a man has sex with twelve women without discharge of semen, he can luster in the complexion until very old; if he has sex with ninety-three women without discharge of semen, he can live a very long life.

凡精少则病，精尽则死。不可不忍，不可不慎。数交而时一泄，精气随长，不能使人虚损。若数交接则泻精，精不得长益，则行精尽矣。在家所以数数交接者，一动不泻，则赢得一泄之精，减即不能数交接。但一月辄再泻精，精气亦自然生长，但迟微不能速起，不如数交接不泻之速也（采女者，少得道，知养性，年一百七十岁，视如十五。殷王奉事之年，问道于彭祖也）。

Generally speaking, if a man holds little semen, he will get sick, and if the semen runs out, he will die. Thus, it is important to restrain oneself in sex and people must be cautious. Multiple intercourse with few discharges will not cause damage to people because semen will be produced quickly, while multiple intercourse with repeated discharges will eventually run out of semen because semen cannot be produced quickly. For those who have sex frequently at home, they can preserve semen without repeated discharge. For those who discharge repeatedly, they should not have sex oftentimes. The semen will grow naturally and slowly for those who discharge twice a month, although it is not as fast as those who have sex without repeated discharge. （Cai Nü, who was enlightened and knew health preservation, lived to 170 years old. However, she looked like a 15-year-old girl. She asked Peng Zu about the method of health preservation when King Yin was in power.）

彭祖曰：奸淫所以使人不寿者，非是鬼神所为也，直由用意俗猥，精动欲泄，务副彼心，竭力无厌，不以相生，反以相害，或惊狂消渴，或癫痴恶疮，为失精之故。但泻辄导引，以补其处。不尔，血脉髓脑日损，风湿犯之，则生疾病，由俗人不知补泻之宜故也。

Peng Zu says: Excessive intercourse makes people not live long, which is not caused by ghosts or gods, but because they often think

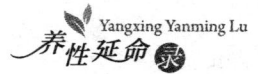

about vulgar and obscene things, leading to the impulse of discharging semen. Every time people indulge themselves in the desire to discharge or even exhaust semen without abstinence, this is harmful rather than beneficial to health, leading to fright epilepsy, mania, consumptive thirst and sore due to insufficient semen. Thus, it is important to conduct the body after discharge every time, so as to tonify the lost semen. Otherwise, blood, vessels, brain and marrow will be damaged day by day, and thus pathogenic wind and dampness will invade the body and cause diseases. This is because ordinary people don't know the appropriate methods of tonification and discharge.

彭祖曰：凡男不可无女，女不可无男。若孤独而思交接者，损人寿，生百病，鬼魅因之共交，失精而一当百。若欲求子，令子长命，贤明富贵，取月宿日施精大佳（月宿日，直录之于后）。

Peng Zu says: A man cannot live without a woman, and vice versa. If a single man always wants to have sex, it will shorten his life span and cause various diseases, and what's more, ghosts take the opportunity to have sex with him. In this case, one ejaculation is equivalent to a hundred times under normal cases. If you want a son and let him live a long life, be wise and rich, it's good to choose the 2nd, 3rd, 5th, 9th and 20th day of every lunar month for sex.

天老曰：人生俱含五常，形法复同，而有尊卑贵贱者，皆由父母合八星阴阳。阴阳不得其时，中也；不合宿，或得其时，人中上也；不合宿，不得其时，则为凡夫矣。合宿交会者，非生子富贵，亦利己身，大吉之兆（八星者，室、参、井、鬼、柳、张、心、斗，月宿在此星，可以合阴阳求子）。

Tian Lao says: Everyone is born with five zang-organs, the same body and physiology, but there are differences in their dignity and status, which all depends on whether the parents meet the eight constellations and Yin-Yang when they have sex. If they do not conform to Yin-Yang, their children will be moderate in talent; if they conform to Yin-Yang rather than constellations, their children will be better than average or superior in talent; if they do not conform to either Yin-Yang or constellations, their children will be ordinary in talent. If they conform to constellations, not only will their children be rich, but also parents can benefit from it, which is a sign of good luck.

月二日、三日、五日、九日、二十日，此是王相生气日，交会各五倍，血气不伤，令人无病。仍以王相日，半夜后，鸡鸣前，徐徐弄玉泉，饮玉浆戏之。若合用春甲寅、乙卯，夏丙午、丁未，

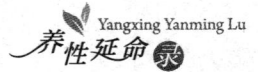

秋庚申、辛酉，冬壬子、癸亥，与上件月宿日合者，尤益佳。若欲求子，待女人月经绝后一日、三日、五日，择中王相日，以气生时，夜半之后乃施精，有子皆男，必有寿贤明。其王相日，谓春甲乙、夏丙丁、秋庚辛、冬壬癸。

The 2nd, 3rd, 5th, 9th and 20th day of each lunar month are King-Minister Days（prime days for sex）. Sexual intercourse five times more than usual does not hurt blood and Qi, or make people sick. People can kiss and play with each other gently and swallow saliva after midnight and before the cockcrow on King-Minister Days. The effect is especially good if Jia Yin and Yi Mao days in spring, Bing Wu and Ding Wei days in summer, Geng Shen and Xin You days in autumn, and Ren Zi and Gui Hai days in winter conform to constellations. If a man wants a son, he can have sex when Yang Qi is exuberant after midnight on the 1st, 3rd and 5th days after a woman's menstruation which coincide with King-Minister Days. The boys must enjoy longevity, virtue and intelligence. King-Minister Days are Jia and Yi days in spring, Bing and Ding days in summer, Geng and Xin days in autumn, and Ren and Gui days in winter.

凡养生，要在于爱精。若能一月再施精，一岁二十四气施精，皆得寿百二十岁。若加药饵，则可长生。所患人年少时不知道，知道亦不能信行；至老乃始知道，便已晚矣，病难养也。虽晚而能自保，犹得延年益寿。若少壮而能行道者，仙可冀矣。

The key to health preservation is to cherish essence and Qi. If a man discharges semen twice a month and 24 times a year, he can enjoy a life of 120 years. If he takes medicine for tonification, he can have his life prolonged. The problem is that people don't know how to preserve sperm when they are young, or they don't follow the rule although they know they should. When they begin to realize the importance in old age, it's too late to recover from the disease. However, it is never too late to preserve semen and people can still prolong life if they follow the rule. If young people can follow the rule, they are very likely to live a long life.

《仙经》曰：男女俱仙之道，深内勿动精，思脐中赤色大如鸡子，乃徐徐出入，精动便退。一旦一夕可数为之，令人益寿。男女各息意共存之，唯须猛念。

*Xianjing（Immortal Classic）*says: The way for both men and women to live long is to insert the penis deeply into the vagina without ejaculating, imagining that there is a red object as big as an egg in the middle of the navel, then move slowly in vagina and stop when semen is stirred. This process can be repeated dozens of times in a day, which

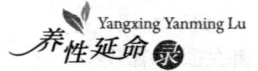

can prolong people's life. Both men and women can prolong life if they have a strong desire to do so.

道人刘京云：春三日一施精，夏及秋一月再施精，冬常闭精勿施。夫天道，冬藏其阳，人能法之，故能长生。冬一施，当春百。

Taoist Liu Jing says: Ejaculate once every three days in spring, twice in a month in summer and autumn, and store semen in winter. The law of nature is to preserve Yang Qi in winter. If people can follow the law, they can live a long life. One ejaculation in winter is equivalent to one hundred ejaculations in spring.

蒯道人言：人年六十便当绝房内。若能接而不施精者，可御女耳。若自度不办者，都远之为上。服药百种，不如此事可得久年也。

Taoist Kuai says: People should completely stop sex at the age of 60. If you can do without ejaculation, you can do it. If you think you can't do, it's better to stay away from sex. Abstinence is better than taking 100 kinds of medicine to make people live longer.

《道林》云：命本者，生命之根本也，决在此道。虽服大药及呼吸导引，备修万道，而不知命之根本。根本者，如树木，但有繁枝茂叶而无根本，不得久活也。

*Daolin* ( *Classic of Tao* ) says: Sex is the foundation of life, which decides whether people can live a long life or not. It makes no sense if people take pills, practice respiratory conduction and strive to practice various health preservation methods, but don't know what the foundation of life is. It's just like a tree, which can't live long if it only has numerous branches and luxuriant leaves without foundation.

命本者，房中之事也。故圣人云：欲得长生，当由所生。房中之事，能生人，能煞人。譬如水火，知用之者，可以养生，不能用之者，立可死矣。交接尤禁醉饱，大忌，损人百倍。欲小便，忍之以交接，令人得淋病，或小便难，茎中痛，小腹强。大恚怒后交接，令人发痈疽。

The foundation of life is sex. So the sage says: If you want to live long, you should do it from this. Sex can not only prolong people's life, but also cause death without abstinence. Just like water and fire. If you know how to use it, you can keep in good health; If you can't use it reasonably, it will even lead to death immediately. It is a taboo to have sex after drinking and eating too much, which can impair people hundredfold. If people have sex while holding their urine, they are prone to gonorrhea, dysuria, penile pain and abdominal distension. If people have sex after great anger, they are prone to carbuncle−abscess.

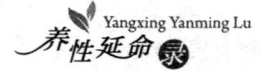

《道机》：房中禁忌，日月晦朔，上下弦望，日月蚀，大风恶雨，地动，雷电，霹雳，大寒暑，春夏秋冬节变之日，送迎五日之中，不行阴阳。本命行年月日，忌禁之尤重（阴阳交错不可合，损血气，泻正纳邪，所伤正气甚矣，戒之）。新沐头，新行疲倦，大喜怒，皆不可行房室。

*Daoji*（*Secret of Tao*）says: The forbidden time for sex is: the 1st, 8th, 9th,15th, 22th, 23th and the last day of a lunar month, eclipse of the sun and moon, the day of strong wind and heavy storm, earthquake, thunder, lightning and thunderbolt, and extremely cold or hot days. People should not have sex on the intersection of the four seasons, five days before and after the summer and winter solstice, and especially the above days of the recurrent year in the twelve−year cycle（Do not have sex when Yin and Yang are in disorder, or it damages Qi and blood, dissipates healthy qi and invites pathogenic Qi）. Besides, people should not have sex right after washing head, or when they are too tired after traveling, or when they are very happy and angry.

彭祖曰：消息之情，不可不知也。又须当避大寒、大热、大雨、大雪、日月蚀、地动、雷震，此是天忌也。醉饱、喜怒、忧愁、悲哀、恐惧，此人忌也。山川神祇、社稷井灶之处，此为地忌也。既避此三忌，又有吉日，春甲乙、夏丙丁、秋庚辛、冬壬癸、四季之月戊已，皆王相之日也。宜用嘉会，令人长生，有子必寿。其犯此忌，既致疾，生子亦凶夭短命。

Peng Zu says: We have to understand the changes of Yin and Yang in the four seasons. When having sex, people must avoid the cold, heat, heavy rain, solar eclipse, lunar eclipse, earthquake and thunder, which are taboos in terms of climate; people must avoid being drunk and full, overjoy, anger, worry, sorrow, fear, which are taboos in terms of people themselves; people must avoid mountains, rivers, places to worship the god of the land and grain, and side of wells and stoves, which are taboos in terms of geographical factors. The three kinds of taboos should be avoided when having sex, and auspicious days are also preferred, i.e. King−Minister Days−Jia and Yi days in spring, Bing and Ding days in summer, Geng and Xin days in autumn, Ren and Gui days in winter, and Wu and Ji days of the four seasons. It is appropriate to have sex on those auspicious days, which can make people live long and have their children's life prolonged if the wife gets pregnant. Violation of these taboos can invite disease or even shorten the life of children.

老子曰：还精补脑，可得不老矣。

Lao Tzu says: Maintaining original spirit can help to prolong life.

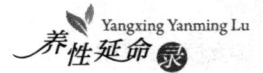

《子都经》曰：施泻之法，须当弱入强出（何谓弱入强出，纳玉茎于琴弦麦齿之间，及洪大便出之，弱纳之，是渭弱入强出。消息之，令满八十动，则阳数备，即为妙也）。

*Zidu Jing*（*Zidu Classic*）says: The method of sex is to put in when weak and pull out when erectile（It means to insert the penis into the vagina when penis is in the state of weakness and pull out when it is erect. Estimate the number and it will be excellent to have 80 movements）.

老子曰：弱入强出，知生之术；强入弱出，良命乃卒。此之谓也。

Lao Tzu says: Inserting when weak and pulling out when erectile is the method of health preservation; if doing it the other way round, even a strong man will be in poor health soon. That's the truth.